Forbidden Emotions—The Key to Healing

Forbidden Emotions—The Key to Healing

By Marti Murphy

ISBN: 978-1-733-52649-4 (Paperback)
ISBN: 978-1-734-35530-7 (eBook)

Library of Congress Control Number: 2020938193
Printed by Ingramspark, in the United States of America.

First printing edition 2020

JEBWizard Publishing
37 Park Forest Rd.
Cranston, RI 02920

www.jebwizardpublishing.com

Table of Contents

Introduction i

    Stuck in a Cycle of Failing ii

    The Moment It All Changed iv

    My Message of Hope for You vii

Living a Liberated Life .... - 1 -

    The Before Picture .... - 1 -

    Chapter Summary 32

Thoughts and Voices 34

    Pay Attention to Your Thoughts 34

    Chapter Summary 60

On Feeling Fully 61

    What Does It Mean to Feel Fully? 61

    Chapter Summary 84

Forbidden Emotions 85

    What Are Forbidden Emotions? 85

    Physical Signs of Forbidden Emotions 85

    Chapter Summary 116

The Basics of Tapping 117

    Chapter Summary 157

Rant Tapping 158

    (AKA "Fuck You" Tapping) 158

    Chapter Summary 194

Argue Tapping 195

    What Is Argue Tapping? 195

Chapter Summary 219

Lifelong Process 220

Chapter Summary 235

Conclusion 236

Acknowledgements 240

About Marti Murphy 242

References 243

End Notes 246

Introduction

I spent first grade in terror of my teacher; taught to believe this nun was God-like. If she were God-like then I knew God was an asshole, and I would burn in hell if I ever said that out loud.

Some days, I would hold a heating pad on my forehead and then tell my mother I did not feel well. She would feel my burning forehead and let me stay home. Relieved, I looked forward to watching The Price Is Right and relaxing on the couch.

My teacher punished us for even the smallest offenses, like leaving our desk open a second longer than she deemed acceptable. If someone had to go to the bathroom, she often told them to wait until class was over. A few of my classmates wet their pants while sitting at their desks because they could not hold it any longer. As punishment, the teacher would grab the offending student, pull their pants down and beat their bare bottom with a wooden ruler until welts appeared and tears rolled down their face.

One day, our teacher was barking orders at us, like she always did. I was so tired of being barked at and bullied, so tired of watching my classmates be terrorized and humiliated.

We were to put our books in our desk, close the lid and fold our hands together on top of the desk within 15 seconds. In an act of pure defiance, I took my two index fingers and slid them under my closed desk lid right in front of her.

Her voice was so calm it was eerie. She told me to come up and stand in front of the room and put my hands out, palms up. She took out her weapon of mass destruction—a wooden ruler— using it on the bodies and psyches of her students. She beat my hands so viciously that at one point I pulled them away because it hurt so much.

In an icy, calm voice she hissed at me, "I am not done with you yet. Put your hands back up here."

I did and braced myself. Tears flowed from my eyes as she thundered away on my palms. By the time she finished, I had welts on my hands that did not allow me to hold a pencil or pick up anything without grimacing.

As you might imagine, faking sick so I could stay home alone with my mom felt a lot safer in the daytime hours.

Nighttime was a different story. My parents often ended up in epic battles that would have my sisters and me quaking in our beds, not able to sleep due to the intense shouting.

I was only six years old, but a part of my brain knew something about all of this was not right. There had to be something more to life than this.

Stuck in a Cycle of Failing

I have been afraid most of my life, having learned at a precious 6 years of age that the world was a very scary place. Fear and anxiety were my dominant emotions.

This thought pattern ran my entire life and was one of the main reasons I was stuck in a cycle of failing for decades. Believing the world is a scary place and living with fear as a constant companion does not help one to take big risks or to trust in a benevolent universe, especially when the first religious person you experience is terrifying and unsafe. Hence, the nun from first grade who was a master in delivering psychic wounding to 6-year-olds.

My fear also meant that I always worked hard to be the good girl. I always tried to get it right, hoping that way I would avoid severe punishments. This was my daily life as a child. The fear and this role of the good girl became so ingrained in me it spilled into my adult years.

I was the good employee—always the responsible and reliable one, stuck between these two parentheses I would place around my life; the learned limits I placed around myself. There was no room for trial and error, no room for mistakes, no room for creativity. I colored inside the safety of those lines, and I lived in quiet desperation, slowly suffocating. Mostly, I tried hard to do what I was told I should do.

Yet an inner voice kept surfacing.

"There's got to be more to life than this."

Before I continue, it is important for you to know this: your inner voice will return again and again and again to help guide you toward choosing you; to help you believe you are worthy of a good life; to help you find your own song.

It may not feel good in the moment you are thinking it, but as you open to it, you learn to be kinder to yourself. When you learn to treat yourself with more kindness, you will see this inner voice is not there to make you feel bad about your choices it is actually calling you home to yourself. It is encouraging you to listen to the guidance that comes from within you. The guidance that is meant to uplift you and thus help wake you up from the nightmare of limitation you have learned to believe is the truth but is not.

Back to my story.

I would hear this voice and, using my non-surrendering will because I did not know better, I would mount my internal forces (forces being an important word here) looking for "that thing" that would turn it all around for me.

I was surrendering nothing, so I would find what I thought was "that thing" and go for it with excitement and gusto, pumping up my ego, but before I knew it, I would seem to hit an invisible barrier. I faded quickly and gave up. I was confounded as to why I could never cross that ever elusive finish line I so wanted to cross. Remember I was using my will to find an answer.

> *"Most men live lives of quiet desperation*
> *and die with their song still inside them."*
>
> *~ Henry David Thoreau*

When I first heard this quote, I thought, "How did Thoreau know?"

I was one of the quiet ones with a song I wanted to sing, but I could not seem to sing it.

I would marvel at bold people—the risk-takers of the world. The ones who would apply for jobs that required more experience than they had. When I would ask them how they had the confidence to stretch themselves in this way, they would say, "I know I'll figure it out once I get my foot in the door." This floored me.

I constantly downplayed myself and my abilities. God forbid if someone had higher expectations of me because what if I couldn't live up to their expectations? I would be devastated and ashamed. So, there I was, coloring inside the lines, unaware of my self-imposed parentheses, living in quiet desperation, living a half-assed version of my life.

As I got older, some things shifted. My life morphed into an okay, mediocre life, but the nagging feeling of "there's got to be more to life than this" persisted.

The Moment It All Changed

Fast forward to New Year's Eve of 2010. While many people were out partying, I sat at home alone. How had another year passed with nothing in my life changing?

I was quietly—desperately—longing for a life I felt happy and excited about. I knew I had to change things, or I would end up as someone filled with regret at the end of their life.

That night, I set my intention to the universe. One of two things had to happen: if there was something out there that would help me change my life, I wanted it to drop into my lap, and if not, then I wanted peace with my mediocre life.

What I know now is this was a genuine moment of surrender for me. I was exhausted from "trying" so hard. With all of my trying, I was not trusting. I was terrified that I was in a game I was always losing, yet out of pure exhaustion and exasperation, I surrendered. I had no clue how or even if things would change. It did not matter in that moment. I just knew where I got myself with my efforts, and I wondered if it were possible not to do it all on my own anymore.

Two weeks later, I found Emotional Freedom Techniques (EFT), also known as Tapping. I found it by following my own internal impulses. I was no longer in my own way. I was open to guidance without even realizing it.

As I look back now, it seems magical the way I found it. I had been guided to the "thing" that would help me change my life and change my life it did.

Little did I know when I started this journey that stuck emotion was to blame for the thoughts I had about myself.

My thoughts were actually lying to me, limiting beliefs about myself, yet felt absolutely true. A few of these thoughts were, you are just a girl, you do not have what it takes. There's something wrong with you. You need to suffer in this life to be worthy or deserving and so many more. These beliefs stopped me from allowing myself to enjoy a life I loved and could feel good about.

It was freeing to realize that the only thing that has ever been "wrong" with me was that I downloaded a set of limiting beliefs as a child that kept me from living a full, rich life.

It is not that I do not feel afraid, anxious, angry or make mistakes anymore, but now I can own and embrace these feelings. I can see these emotions as signs that I'm listening to and believing limiting beliefs, which takes me out of alignment with my true self. I then feel through my emotions (with processes I have developed), and I am able to move forward with more self-compassion and understanding.

It is a funny thing, but the more self-compassion and understanding you have for yourself, and others, the better your life gets.

My Message of Hope for You

Fast forward to my life now.

I left my corporate career and started a personal development business. I became a Certified EFT Practitioner which, in the past, I would have self-sabotaged. I would have become too afraid to move forward, but helped by EFT, I did not sabotage myself.

My inspiration to assist others came from my own previous feelings of being stuck. I thought if anyone had ever felt as stuck as I had, and I could help them, then I wanted to help them move beyond self-limiting behaviors.

Finding Tapping has changed my life, and it continues to change it for the better. Now I have a surprising, slightly strange, yet highly effective technique literally at my fingertips. How simple is that? When I feel the push to go backward, to color inside the lines, I use this technique to keep me moving forward. I am a work in progress—we all are—but now I have a technique that can help me along this journey.

This is my message of hope for you.

If you feel stuck in your life. If you hear that inner voice saying, "There's got to be more." If you have a song to sing, yet feel clueless as to what that song is, hang on, because you are in for a ride. A ride that can be truly transformational, and help you feel better about yourself. A ride that can help you remember the truth of who you are. An infinite, capable, amazing human.

You can become the awe-inspiring person your dog thinks you are. You can become the person you have dreamed about becoming. You can become the person you see in someone else.

Because the truth is you already are the awe-inspiring person your dog thinks you are. You already are the person you have dreamed about becoming. You already are the person you see in someone else.

You just need some help uncovering that person. And I am here to help you.

You are your own guru.

You are the most important person in your life.

You can find that something more you have been longing for.

You can feel good about you, and you can create a life you desire.

You can learn to embrace this amazing, full palette of emotions you were born with.

You can find these emotions have the power to change you and your life.

You can reignite the Divine spark within you.

This book is dedicated to everyone who learned that their feelings are wrong, bad, or should be denied or pushed through quickly.

It is my firm belief there would be a lot less blind fury, prejudice, domestic abuse, animal abuse, road rage, poverty, and obesity if we were all allowed, even encouraged, to feel fully in a safe and healthy way. To embrace the full spectrum of emotions we are all gifted with.

Emotions are not the problem. Emotions are indicators to us of our state of being. The challenge is that most of us learned early in life to suppress our instinct to feel. Many of us were taught to be seen and not heard, or that as a kid what we think, and feel does not matter. We were told how to feel and how to behave and to suppress what came naturally. As children, we were forced to sit all day in school and were bombarded with relatively useless information. On top of it all, we were taught we must get certain grades to matter or excel in the material world.

If we as children were encouraged to trust ourselves and could say what we think and feel what we feel, I believe we would all see that we are equal inhabitants of this amazing planet we share. The planet would be healthier too, because the people inhabiting it would be healthier mentally, emotionally, physically, and spiritually. The planet is a representation of what is happening inside the collective consciousness of humanity. The suppression of emotion is what leads to inappropriate actions, with people harming others, harming animals, and harming the planet.

This book is about hope. When you learn a healthy, safe way to work through buried or suppressed memories, you can liberate yourself from the emotional blocks that cause havoc in your life.

How to feel fully, in a safe and healthy way, is what I outline in this book.

I hope that, if you are drawn to read this book, you will find faith in there being a better way and, in embracing this better way. You will be liberated from the emotions that keep you stuck in any area of your life.

It is also my belief that as you embrace, accept, and feel all your emotions, you will release negative emotions frozen in your body and mind. You will discover that you not only feel better but that your "resting thought rate" (which I will explain later) is infinitely more positive. Being in a positive state of being assists you in creating a life you love.

A life where you wake up and feel excited about what is to come. A life where you appreciate what you have, and positive expectation for what comes next. You will discover the perfect formula for creating a life that lights you up. When you live this way, you are doing the best thing you can for yourself.

Once you learn how to feel fully, you can continue through your life with more confidence in yourself. This will be demonstrated in your day-to-day life experiences. It is not that you will be free of challenges, but you will learn to handle challenges far more effectively and with confidence.

I like to say it this way: you will feel empowered and clearer about what is best for you and your life, and the decisions you make will reflect this.

You will remember who you are and be more connected to Source, God, the Universe, Higher Self, better emotional intelligence, or whatever word resonates with you regarding this.

If you have felt stuck in a cycle of failing, ask yourself: What if failing is the key to something greater than I ever imagined?

This book comes from years of personal work and countless hours working with clients, whose names have been changed in this book, from all walks of life and all over the world. It reveals the common thread within each person and the primary reason we do not move forward in our lives.

Wishing you the best on your journey,

Marti Murphy

Living a Liberated Life

The Before Picture

You are a smart, driven, responsible person. If you get honest with yourself, you will say your life's not bad, but it does not feel good either. There are times, especially in the wee hours of the morning when you wake up and can't go back to sleep, that something inside of you just knows "there's got to be more." In these moments of longing, you feel that somehow, you are missing the boat, but you are not sure where the boat is or, if you found it, how to board it.

You think you've found "that thing" and get excited trying to create this elusive "more." You might even make some progress, but before you know it, despite your best efforts, you are back to square one and telling yourself, "my life is not that bad" until you hear about friends or acquaintances building their dream home, or who just retired and are traveling the world, or are moving to a new exotic place to start a new adventure or more importantly those who seem to be fulfilled, despite whatever worldly possessions or achievements they have or don't have.

You want to feel happy for them, but all you can do is feign excitement because deep down you are envious. It is in these moments you fall back into this place of longing for more. What appears to be their good fortune hammers home the feeling that you are just settling and that something must be missing within you to not be living a life that you desire; one you have actually chosen for yourself, despite what family or society says you should want.

This feeling slowly chips away your self-esteem. Deep down you feel a quiet desperation, like a slow death of your spirit. Your situation is not bad enough, and yet it is not good enough, either. You feel stuck, and it is as if parentheses have been placed around your life and you cannot move beyond them—you can spend decades in this place of limbo.

I have felt this way.

That you could lead a fulfilling life—and a life not measured by the success model that most of us have been enculturated to measure ourselves by—feels more elusive than ever. (It is important to note here that to learn to measure yourself from your own standards that come from your heart, mind and soul is true freedom no matter what anyone else thinks.)

Without creating our own standard of what success means to you, you are trapped in a maze where it seems like there's a club for "those people" who seem to have this magical membership to a wildly successful life and you are not a part of it. You hear about it all the time, and now you long for a membership. You long for a life that feels so out of reach to you, and you long for liberation.

What Does It Mean to Live a Liberated Life?

The After Picture

Your liberation starts something like this: You notice you are releasing behaviors that were not serving you because they were limiting you.

Below are examples of behaviors I had that I released with tapping. Do any of them apply to you? If so, you will release them after you tap.

Comparing Yourself to Others

This was the first behavior I noticed I stopped doing after I tapped. About three months into tapping, I realized that I was no longer making these crazy comparisons that left me feeling worse about myself, such as comparing my life with movie stars like Julia Roberts and Reese Witherspoon. The funniest part of these comparisons is that I have never wanted to be an actress, but I still chose impossible comparisons that left me losing big time. I was so caught up in the consciousness of better than or less than.

I was in an online workshop where the topic was about what happens to you when you compare yourself with others. One of the instructors said, "Whenever you compare yourself to someone else, you always lose." She said that most of us make the comparison where we feel "less than," which can leave us feeling like a loser. Even if you compare and place yourself on top, that never feels good because it is outwardly directed.

When you are outwardly directed, you are actually allowing the ego—the bully in your brain which I will discuss later—to run your show. When you allow the ego to run your show, it is a step up for fear and anxiety.

What happens when you are "winning" and then something doesn't go your way?

What happens when some goals you have don't become realized?

Notice how you feel then and what your self-talk sounds like. It is usually self-defeating. It often sounds like you have done something wrong, or you are not thinking about this positively enough. There's often a self-blaming reason you are not enough.

Who do you compare yourself to?

When you release pent-up emotions with tapping, you will notice comparing yourself to others becomes a thing of the past the more you catch yourself in the act of doing this.

Negative Thinking

This encompassed my general view of things. One of the best things I did for myself was to stop watching the news. Before making this decision, I watched the news every night just before going to bed. The majority of what is being reported is highly negative; it is a constant bombardment of what is not working in your city or town, the country, and the world.

When I fell asleep, these negative stories stewed in my brain all night long. With this constant negativity, not surprisingly, people lament about the world going to "hell in a handbasket." Some people might argue "you should stay informed," but did it add to my life to stay informed and hear all the stories of what is not working? No, it took away from my peace of mind. After I stopped watching the news, I found this change had an immediate effect on decreasing my negative thinking.

What negative thoughts stew in your brain, and where do they come from?

When you release pent-up emotions with tapping, you will notice your resting thought rate is infinitely more positive.

Self-criticism

This goes hand in hand with negative thinking, but it is directed exclusively at yourself. It is your negative view of yourself; what you say to yourself about how things might turn out for you.

When you hear yourself saying things like, "With my luck, it will not turn out," think about what you are anchoring onto your psyche with that statement. You essentially say that no matter what you do, things more than likely will not work out for you. Check the results you are getting in any area of your life, and this will tell you a lot about your thinking. When things are not where you want them to be, that is an indicator that your thoughts about this subject are not serving you.

What negative thoughts do you have about yourself?

When you release pent-up emotions with tapping, you will notice you become more compassionate with yourself and less self-critical.

Being Critical of Others

Judging others seems to come so naturally to most of us. We make judgments about people, situations, places, and things all the time. You can easily see the worst in people. Thus, paying attention to your thoughts can be very eye-opening.

What do you criticize in others?

With tapping you will notice that you are a lot more compassionate of others' behaviors in the after picture.

Not Reacting as Quickly

When someone or something triggers a rapid-fire emotional response in you, it is easy to react before thinking about it. For example, when you feel judged by someone, it can light you up like a pinball machine. What I mean by this, is the physiology of your body gets activated when we feel stress because of a reaction we have to someone's judgment of us, cortisol levels rise in the body.

When you have elevated levels of cortisol—often called the "stress hormone"—your body perceives this stress and your adrenal glands make and release cortisol into your bloodstream. This elevated cortisol causes an increase in your heart rate and blood pressure. When this happens, digestion slows along with your ability to reason because blood flows away from your prefrontal cortex, the thinking, reasoning, and creative part of the brain. The prefrontal cortex is the slower part of the brain. Without access to this part of the brain you can become more reactive than reasonable because of the elevated level of cortisol.

When you are in pure reaction mode, you lose your ability to think and speak rationally; your emotions get the best of you. This is said best by Leadership Master Coach, Blair Singer, who said: "When emotions get high, intelligence gets low."

Reacting quickly and without thought is often related to the fight-or-flight response. Something happens that makes you feel threatened. You want to fight, or you want to run. It is a primal reaction to keep us safe.

What triggers a rapid-fire emotional response in you?

Tapping helps calm the fight-or-flight response and helps you to think instead of just reacting, which gives you the space and time to come up with better solutions.

Overreacting

One time I was at a storage unit unpacking a box of table lighting packed with Styrofoam peanuts. It was a breezy day and these foam peanuts were spewing all over the place. When I opened the box, it was as if these peanuts multiplied. They were sticking to my pant legs and my jacket and, suddenly, I felt overwhelming anger. With arms flailing, I swatted at these foam peanuts and cursed at them as if they were attacking me— like they had it out for me. Had someone seen me, they would have turned around and walked as fast as they could in the opposite direction. I was in fight-mode. When I calmed myself down, I realized how over-the-top my reaction had been, a clear indicator I had a lot of pent-up emotion.

Have you overreacted lately? What stresses you out?

When you manage your stress and release more pent-up emotion with tapping, you will find you overreact less and less.

These are some behaviors I have seen major progress in within myself. What behaviors would you like to shift?

How to Tell You are on the Right Path

When you release the stuck emotions that do not serve you, you notice this new and improved version of yourself emerging. Exciting opportunities seem to come your way, and you embrace them with a calm assuredness that feels new to you.

You notice you are gaining positive traction long past where you previously would have self-sabotaged. You feel more hopeful and have more positive expectations. You notice you are feeling better about yourself and your life.

You notice positive changes in many areas of your life: your relationships are smoother, your job feels easier, your financial life improves, and your health improves. You notice that many things that would have bothered you before no longer bother you. Self-sabotage becomes something you recognize and overcome with regularity, and you live a more consciously aware life. It is not that negative thinking and behaviors are eliminated from your life—you are human —but now you can work through them and release the learned limits you've placed on yourself.

Here is a real bonus: As you get in touch with what you desire, that elusive "thing" you have longed for no longer exists because you like the person you are. Your life feels better all the way around because you are feeling better.

You will hear family and friends say things to you like:

"I can't put my finger on it, but there's something different about you."

"Have you done something different? You look happier."

"Did you lose weight? You look really good."

They see outward evidence of the internal changes you are making. That is why they cannot put their finger on it; energetically, you are different, and that is what they are picking up on.

Your life works for you, and you cannot always put your finger on it, either, other than just knowing you feel better. Is feeling better the thing you want? Why do you want the things you want (the new home, the loving relationship, the new job, more money)? If you think about this, you want these things because of the feeling you will have in possessing. You want to feel good. What also can happen is the material things you have longed for can become things you can take or leave without the need to have them. This is real freedom. This creates space for new possibilities to come to you that are greater than you've been able to imagine.

Living a liberated life is being true to yourself because you are getting in touch with what you think and feel. You care for the most important person in your life—you. You have liberated yourself from the suffocating feeling that you have missed the boat.

Living a liberated life means that you are feeling fully from this amazing palette of emotions you came into this world with—you are feeling your life.

When you allow yourself to feel what you are feeling in any moment, and this means anything on the spectrum from hatred, jealousy, rage and frustration to contentment, peace, and joy, you are allowing it all. No emotion is off limits to you anymore. There is no such thing as a forbidden emotion because you just feel them and allow them to move through you. (I have devoted an entire chapter to talk about Forbidden Emotions, so more on that later.)

By allowing yourself to feel the forbidden emotions—on your own, in a safe place—you do not need to act on them. When you allow them to be, you live more fully. When you become more present in each moment, you rekindle your creative mind. When your creative mind is rekindled, your ability to hear your intuition grows. When you trust your intuition, you make life choices in your own best interest. You notice your life looks like something you desire and, perhaps, more important, something you allow to be designed through you. You stop asking yourself to be someone you are not and stop living in a way that is not congruent for you.

When you allow yourself to feel the forbidden emotions, you get clear on whether you need to express or act on these emotions. You become clear about who you are and how to live your life.

There's a great line from the movie *Out of Africa* where Robert Redford's character, Denys Finch Hatton, says to Karen Blixen:

"I don't want to find out one day that I'm at the end of someone else's life."

This line says it well.

The Ninety Second Movement of Emotions

I heard an interview with *Quantum Success* coach Christy Whitman. She said an emotion takes ninety seconds to move through us. I will add that an unencumbered emotion takes ninety seconds to move through us. An emotion we do not avoid, bury, or stop takes ninety seconds to move through us.

I did an experiment to check this out for myself. When I would feel a strong emotion, such as anger, I would first use EFT and allow myself to express whatever I was pissed off about. I would Rant Tap—I will teach you this later—and just talk out loud, spew out whatever I needed to get off my chest, tapping while I did so.

This released a lot of the stuck energy I had around the emotion of anger. Using tapping when you feel a strong emotion is an important lifelong practice because the cumulative effect is profound.

This is what I mean by unencumbered, and this is how you can unblock your emotions. When you feel an emotion, instead of blocking it, if you just allow it to move through you in this way, you might notice it does take around ninety seconds. Rant tapping was key for me to free myself from suppressed emotions. Anger, for example, was a big one for me. Once I allowed myself to free myself from years of suppressed anger, when I would feel anger in an unencumbered way, it moved through me in around ninety seconds.

I have noticed that emotions are like waves. As you allow them to move through you without resisting them, they build up like waves. Here is how it works: Something happens, and you feel an emotion build and crescendo as if crashing up against the shore, and then it dissipates. A particular emotion might continue to move through you in waves, but when left to its own natural rhythm, it will fade away the more you allow yourself to feel it. I do find these waves of emotions come in ninety second intervals when allowed.

I suggest you start thinking of all emotions as waves; when they start to build, instead of burying them, tap through them to release them, as well as the buildup of buried emotions you have accumulated over the years. You will notice that, over time, they do what they should do: move through you.

Thoughts Generate Emotions, Which Create Beliefs

Let's talk about how your thoughts generate your emotions: a thought creates an emotional response.

Here is the simple formula.

Your Thoughts → Create Your Emotions → Create Your Beliefs

What is a thought, really? According to neuroscience, a thought is the process of an electrical impulse in your brain that stimulates some part of it, prompting another electrical impulse. This sequence of electrical impulses is what we call thinking. A thought would then be the electrical impulse that gets wired into your brain. Thoughts themselves get wired into your brain.

In his article, *"Can You Change Your Brain by Thinking Differently," Dr Joe Dispenza says:*

"So, what is it then that talks us out of true change? The answer is: our feelings and our emotions. Feelings and emotions are the end-products of an experience. When we are in the midst of any experience, all of our five senses are gathering sensory data and a rush of information is sent back to the brain through those five different pathways. As this occurs, gangs of neurons will string into place and organize themselves to reflect that event. The moment that these jungles of nerve cells become patterned into networks, they will fire into place and release chemicals. Those chemicals that are released are called emotions.

Emotions and feelings, then, are neurochemical memories of past events. We can remember experiences better when we can recall how they felt. For example, do you remember where you were on 9/11? You probably can clearly recall where you were that day, at that exact time, because you can remember the novel feeling that woke you up enough to pay full attention. More than likely, it was a different feeling than you'd had in a long time."

According to Dr. Joe Dispenza, we create our emotions by the thoughts we think about an experience, and our emotions are by-products of our past experiences.

There's a funny saying by personal development speaker and author Dan Millman.

"What do you think you're thinking, when you think you're not thinking?"

When I started paying attention to the thoughts rumbling around in my head, I was astonished to hear how many of my thoughts were so negative. I felt like I had a cesspool of negative thoughts between my ears. These thoughts had been running the show of my life and, because of them, through self-fulfilling prophecy I had unconsciously created what was showing up in my life for decades. The good news is my unconscious thoughts were becoming conscious, and it is when my thoughts were conscious that I could actually shift them.

Consider this from stem cell Biologist Dr. Bruce Lipton, from his June 7, 2012 article *"The Wisdom of Your Cells."*

"At the university I graduated from conventional microscopes into electron microscopy and had a further opportunity to look into the lives of cells. The lessons I learned profoundly changed my life and gave me insights about the world that I would like to share with you.

Using electron microscopy, I not only saw the cells from the outside, but I went through the cell's anatomy and understand the nature of its organization, its structures, and its functions. As much as people talk about flying into outer space, I was flying into inner space and seeing new vistas, having greater appreciation of life, the nature of cells and our involvement with our own cells.

At this time, I also trained in cell culturing. In about 1968 I cloned stem cells, doing my first cloning experiments under the guidance of Dr. Irv Konigsberg, a brilliant scientist who created the first stem cell cultures.

The stem cells I was working with were called myoblasts. Myo means muscle; blast means progenitor. When I put my cells in the culture dishes with the conditions that support muscle growth, the muscle cells evolved, and I would end up with giant contractile muscles. However, if I changed the environmental situation, the fate of the cells would be altered. I would start off with my same muscle precursors but in an altered environment they would actually form bone cells. If I further altered the conditions, those cells became adipose or fat cells. The results were exciting because while every cell was genetically identical, the fate of the cells was controlled by the environment in which I placed them.

This is powerful to learn that though cells are genetically identical, these cells can change through the environment they were placed in. It begs to question, what environment are you subjecting your cells to and how is this affecting them and what can you do to change the environment your cells get exposed to, so you can change them for the better."

In *"The Intention Experiment: Using Your Thoughts to Change Your Life and the World,"* award-winning journalist and the author, Lynne McTaggart writes:

"A sizable body of research exploring the nature of consciousness, carried on for more than thirty years in prestigious scientific institutions around the world, shows that thoughts are capable of affecting everything from the simplest machines to the most complex living beings. This evidence suggests that human thoughts and intentions are an actual physical "something" with astonishing power to change our world. Every thought we have is tangible energy with the power to transform. A thought is not only a thing; a thought is a thing that influences other things."

Here is another thing to consider about your thoughts from an article by Jordan Lejuwaan on some basic biology, *"How Your Thoughts Program Your Cells"*:

"There are thousands upon thousands of receptors on each cell in our body. When we have feelings of anger, sadness, guilt, excitement, happiness or nervousness, each separate emotion releases its own flurry of neuropeptides. Those peptides surge through the body and connect with those receptors, which change the structure of each cell as a whole. Where this gets interesting is when the cells actually divide. If a cell has been exposed to a certain peptide more than others, the new cell that is produced through its division will have more of the receptor that matches with that specific peptide. Likewise, the cell will also have less receptors for peptides that its mother/sister cell was not exposed to as often."

Here is a study from US National Library of Medicine National Institutes of Health:

The Effect of Emotional Freedom Technique, EFT on Stress Biochemistry: A Randomized Controlled Trial[1]

"This study examined the changes in cortisol levels and psychological distress symptoms of eighty-three nonclinical subjects receiving a single hour-long intervention. Subjects were randomly assigned to either an EFT group, a psychotherapy group receiving supportive interviews or a no treatment group.

Salivary cortisol assays were performed immediately before and 30 minutes after the intervention. Psychological distress symptoms were assessed. The EFT group showed statistically significant improvements in anxiety, depression, the overall severity of symptoms, and symptom breadth. The EFT group experienced a significant decrease in cortisol level compared with the decrease observed in the supportive interviews and no treatment groups. The decrease in cortisol levels in the EFT group mirrored the observed improvement in psychological distress."

Cool, huh? Basically, Dr. Bruce Lipton, Lynne McTaggert, Jordan Lejuwaan, and the authors of the study conducted through the US National Library of Medicine National Institutes of Health are giving hope for change.

In my personal experience I have seen the changes consistent tapping can do. I have seen in my own life and the lives of many clients I have worked with the ability to actually reprogram our negative thought cells to become more optimistic. Tapping is my favorite tool to use to allow changes to occur from within.

When you pay attention to your thoughts, you become conscious of them, and when you know your thoughts, you can use tapping to shift your thoughts. At first, it can feel uncomfortable to be conscious of your thoughts; you may find you want to control them, slay them, extradite them, or stop them.

Thoughts and the emotions tied to those thoughts have the power to create beliefs within us. Simply put:

A belief is a thought you have been thinking over and over again.

You cannot stop a thought you have programmed yourself to think, but if a belief is a thought you have been thinking repeatedly, fair to say that, given some time, you can reprogram the repetitive thoughts you have been thinking and ultimately feel relief and experience positive change.

This makes sense in that after I had been tapping consistently for about ninety days, people pointed out the difference they noticed in me. As I focused on releasing a lot of the negative thoughts I had in place, gradually my thoughts naturally became more positive. Why would this be? I rarely tapped on a positive thought when I started tapping.

My theory is that negative thoughts get programmed into us over the years. I believe that we are all born loaded with positivity. It just gets clouded over through the years as those who raise us and educate us teach us what they were taught, which is often language that places limits on us.

Examples are: You cannot do that. You are not smart enough. You do not want to get disappointed. On and on it goes.

As I freed myself from the high cortisol levels that had flooded my cells for decades, my natural positive mindset resurfaced. Tapping sends a soothing signal to the amygdala which calms the nervous system by lower the cortisol levels in your body. Since cortisol is a stress hormone released by the adrenal glands, it is important in helping your body deal with stressful situations, as your brain triggers its release in response to different stress. The problem is when cortisol levels are too high for too long, this hormone can hurt you more than it helps. I have found tapping to be a highly effective technique I use to calm myself through calming my physiology.

The beauty of tapping is you can now embrace your negative thoughts and no longer fear them. Do not try to stop them. Let's circle back and explore this idea further.

Can You Stop Your Thoughts?

Try and stop a thought. Really try to stop it.

To demonstrate, let's do an exercise. Here goes:

Stop the next thought that comes into your head.

If you think it helps, close your eyes, and try it. Pay close attention. Try to stop the next thought that comes. Stop it. Just stop it. I think I am making my point. Now, you may have had a split second that felt blank, but you cannot stop your thoughts.

You will find you have about as much success at stopping your thoughts as you would if I asked you to go to the ocean shore and hold back the tide.

I will give you a personal example: I was raised in a devout Catholic family. I often thought that my father would have done well as a priest because he did his best to follow the dogma of Catholicism to the letter. He preached it incessantly, and I absorbed it all like a sponge. I was terrified that if I did not behave a certain way and if I entertained certain thoughts that were less than holy, I would spend my life in the hereafter with the devil as my companion, burning in the eternal flames of hell. These thoughts sucked.

One time, in my early teens, I was in church and the priest used the phrase, "Jesus is coming." My mind immediately produced a very sexual thought about this. Mortified, I was convinced that, because of that thought, I would burn in hell.

I believed it was my fault I did not control this "sinful" thought. I believed my fate was sealed because of "inappropriate" thoughts like these.

I could've thrown in the towel and lived a life of hedonism. I mean, why not? I was headed to hell anyway. But I kept trying to control my thoughts; I kept trying to be a "good girl." I clung to the hope that somehow, some way, I could repent, be forgiven and be saved.

The problem was I kept thinking sinful thoughts, thoughts I believed should not enter my head. I was not able to stop my thoughts, and this terrified me.

The more I felt pressured to not think those thoughts, the more they invaded my brain, as if they had a mind of their own.

I was in chronic fight-or-flight mode, so my ability to think rationally was limited. If I would have had my senses about me, I might have realized that I knew no one who was getting this stuff right; if I did end up in hell, I would know a lot of the people there. I did not make that connection until my twenties because my programming was so deeply entrenched.

How to Bypass Unhelpful Thoughts

So, what can you do if you can't stop your thoughts?

I am not just talking about what I thought was lewd back when I was a teenager. I'm talking about any thoughts you do not like— thoughts you think are unacceptable to think. Maybe you have thoughts of revenge for someone you felt hurt by. Maybe you feel hatred toward someone, and you tell yourself you should not feel this way. Maybe you are stressed out and afraid on the job and you fear you will be fired. Maybe you want your ex to suffer as you have. These kinds of thoughts.

How can you deal with this inability to stop these thoughts? Here is the solution:

You cannot stop a thought, but you can interrupt it.

So often when I tell clients this, a look of relief will wash over their faces. For many, it creates a paradigm shift; it takes the pressure off of thinking you can actually stop your thoughts. When you accept the thoughts and learn how to quiet them down, it releases the inner battle of the thoughts. Once you have done this a few times, you recognize when the argumentative thoughts go into battle again.

If you check in with yourself, I will wager that, if you go back through your past, you have bullied yourself for thinking certain dark thoughts. The odds are high that you are still bullying yourself.

Dark Thoughts Create Dark Emotions

Years ago, I was talking to a friend who was going through a rough time with a girlfriend. Shit was hitting the fan for him. He told me how dark thoughts would crop up and it troubled him. The reason I call them dark is because that is how they feel to most of us when we feel them. You will see what I mean.

He was experiencing violent thoughts about what he would like to do to his girlfriend's ex-husband. The thoughts were so uncomfortable that he shook his head trying to shake these thoughts out of his mind. He had no luck with this technique. I have tried this strategy, also with no success.

This bears repeating. You cannot stop your thoughts, but you can interrupt them.

Another way to describe dark thoughts is the thoughts you try to resist thinking. These are forbidden on some level for you, and they make you feel bad about yourself for even thinking them.

I will define dark thoughts as any thoughts you feel ashamed or embarrassed about. You would love to extract them from your mind. You would prefer you did not have them because they make you feel like there's something wrong with you.

Beating the "Bully in Your Brain"

So, how are dark thoughts delivered to you?

You may be wondering what this means, but I find dark thoughts come from what I call the "Bully in Your Brain." I will discuss this more in depth in the next chapter. For now, let's just say that the Bully in Your Brain delivers these thoughts with a heap of judgment. This is otherwise known as your inner critic or your ego. It is the voice in your head that serves up thoughts that leave you thinking and then feeling, for example:

"I'm not good enough."

"I don't have what it takes."

"I'm too old."

"I'm too young."

"I can't do that."

"I'm not a good person."

On and on ad nauseam, these limiting beliefs run the show behind the scenes in your unconscious. Without realizing it, you put a limit on what is possible for you. These thoughts end up in a loop in your head. It is like watching the clothes in a dryer tumbling, only you are hearing the same thoughts tumbling around and around until you are left feeling horrible about yourself. This goes back to the article, *"How Your Thoughts Program Your Cells,"* you have unconsciously programmed your cells to create more negative thoughts.

We do not like going to a dark place and feeling bad. It is uncomfortable to feel bad, and it is uncomfortable to notice dark thoughts because they create feelings that just do not feel good.

Have you ever died from an emotion?

It might feel like you have come close, but if you are reading this book now then you are alive, feeling an unpleasant emotion has not killed you. One key to dealing with dark, self-critical thoughts—something I have found repeatedly to be true for me and my clients—is to notice if you are judging yourself for these dark thoughts. Often you have to pay attention to notice the judgment.

When I am working with my clients, I notice how often self-judgment surfaces and I find this is a critical part of the healing journey. When you recognize your own self-judgment, you are then in the power seat to release it. This is a lifelong practice for all of us. When you see it, you can use tapping to acknowledge and release it.

To be clear about what I consider dark thoughts, they sound like the following.

"There's something really wrong with me."

"I'm just too fucked up."

"I'm way too lazy."

"I'm a fat pig."

"I'm a loser."

"I'm a failure."

"I should be ashamed of myself."

Here are sneaky versions:

"I know better and I did it anyway."

"What was I thinking?"

"I shouldn't have said that."

"I walked into that one."

"I should do that."

The above are relatively clear. Some are sneakier. Here is one I find interesting.

"What's better, the devil I know or the devil I don't know?"

This self-limiting thought suggests that you have only two choices: what is not working well for you or something even worse than what you have now.

What about a third option? What about the option that there's something better for you?

These sneakier thoughts, which appear to be a milder version of dark thoughts, are just as effective in rendering you incapable of moving forward past a certain point. They also leave you feeling bad, and when you feel bad, how creative and inspired do you think you can be? Therefore, how effective can you be? I think you may know the answers to these questions.

You not only have to be wary of the Bully in Your Brain, but you may run into naysayers disguised as family and friends.

Any time you have a desire to change your life or do something different and you express this to someone else, watch out for a nay-saying message such as:

"You have it made where you're at."

"You've tried this before and failed."

"Why would you want to mess up what you've worked so hard for?"

What you're being told is:

"You have the best you can get right now, so don't reach any higher, because you'll just end up disappointed."

This is can also be a dark thought (being expressed to you) because it is putting a limit on your life and what is possible for you.

Now if you are thinking, *"I cannot just change those thoughts because I have tried and I cannot get rid of them,"* do not worry, I will show you how you can.

Is Crying a Measure of Weakness... or Strength?

I was talking with someone about the death of her father, and she told that her husband realized how strong she was because she never shed a tear. I knew that she, and her husband, considered not crying to be a measure of strength. Please consider that the opposite is true. Feeling grief in all of its discomfort requires great strength. It is a challenging experience to grieve loss. It is challenging to unearth any painful feelings so you can release them, primarily because you were trained to not feel certain emotions.

When I got the phone call from the retirement village where my mother was living, the administrator asked me if I was driving. I said, "Yes, and I know what that means." I knew what was coming. I pulled over, and she dropped the reality bomb. My mother had died.

They had found my mother in her home. I immediately burst into tears. Unfortunately, the administrator had been trained like most of us, and her comment was something like, "You're not going to do your mother any good behaving this way."

I was shocked out of my crying. I stopped immediately. A feeling of incredible anger replaced my grief. I snapped back at her, "My mother's dead. I'm not sure she'd care at this point."

It is the unfortunate way many of us have been trained to view emotions. So, when we are uncomfortable with them, we are naturally uncomfortable with allowing someone else to feel them.

Now what if, when I burst into tears, she had said "That is good my dear, let it all out. The more you feel the more you heal." If she had not been trained to dissociate from emotional outbursts, she could have provided validation and aided in my healing process. This is something I needed to give to myself: validation of my feelings, whether she could or not. The only real freedom I have. The same is true for you.

After my mother passed, my sisters and I attended to the disarray in my mother's home. It was overwhelming because of the way she'd died and what she had left behind. We were all swelling with the suppression of very intense feelings, and we were doing the best we could in trying to cope. With the training—or maybe the lack of training—we'd had in how to cope, sometimes it went well and other times it sucked. Occasionally, a major fight ensued. We were trying to surf a tsunami of emotion with no roadmap or effective skills to assist in processing what was happening within us.

Understanding what I do now I would say that, had we'd been taught how to deal with massive mixtures of emotions, we could've grieved in a much healthier way. Someone close to my family told me we were all a mess because we were freaking out. It was a huge problem for them, and they could not be around us.

They could not handle the way my sisters and I were trying to cope with losing our mother, the way she'd died and the mess we were left to clean up. This scenario had the potential to send the most balanced individual into a tailspin, much less people who were not often ensured that it was okay to feel whatever we feel. I was flabbergasted this family member was blaming their discomfort with the entire situation on my sisters and me, and saying it was because we were a mess.

Looking back now yes, we were a mess! But it was appropriate to be feeling a mess of emotions amidst a messy situation. Pure, raw emotion has no place to hide. At some point an emotional upheaval is a guarantee, and so the circumstances of my mother's death caused an emotional upheaval.

I have realized that our family member was actually dealing with their own unprocessed emotions around the grief they had suffered in their life, with no real genuine release of it. They were not capable of behaving any differently than they had, which is also true for me and my sisters; we were all doing the best we were capable of back then. Since then one of us sisters has passed and I would say that we have all been very open-hearted about her passing and been able to love and support each other through it as we've allowed ourselves our individual expression of our grief and journey through mourning.

When Abnormal Feelings are Completely Normal

Years ago, I remember hearing someone say, *"Feeling what feels abnormal in an abnormal situation is normal."*

What a relief! This was the first time I would ever entertain the idea that when you are in a situation that is unusual, and your feelings feel "abnormal" to you...this is normal. This was enlightening and simple for me to realize. What is actually happening is we are judging emotions as normal or abnormal when emotions are just the emotions.

An example from my own life would be the biblical commandment *"Honor Thy Father and Mother,"* yet I had experiences where my parents, being human, did not behave in a manner that one might deem as honorable, yet I was taught there's no variation on this. So, what are you supposed to feel when a parent behaves dishonorably, or unjustly, and you are told to honor them with no exceptions? Well unexpressed anger grew into rage when hypocrisy is witnessed, and I was not supposed to feel rage. What I have come to understand now, is that my rage was actually a very normal emotion I was taught was abnormal, even forbidden.

It takes practice to believe that whatever you are feeling is okay, and I encourage you to begin practicing sooner rather than later.

Sometimes emotions feel messy, and it is usually because the situation you are in is messy. Given that, doesn't it make sense that messy emotions result from messy situations?

When you learn that certain emotions are off limits, you automatically might think that you need to remove them from the banquet table of emotions that you have been endowed with. But because you cannot remove them, you stuff them down internally and, over time, these emotions build up until they must release. When they do release, it is often done inappropriately. Remember my Styrofoam peanuts example? Case in point.

You think you are calm and peaceful until you get two hangers stuck together and you end up enraged, or you are unpacking a box that has Styrofoam packing peanuts inside and they stick to your shirt and you bat at them wildly and scream.

Or you have had a fight with your spouse, and you are trying not to feel angry when you really do, and you take it out on someone or something else.

Or you are driving down the highway, singing to tunes, and someone cuts you off, and you want to mow them down.

Or your sibling comes to your house and their veins look like they will explode out of their neck, and you attempt to talk to them about their anger. You ask them what is going on and they say nothing because they have learned to suppress their anger. The next thing you know, they are picking at you over seemingly inconsequential things and you punch a wall. They look at you in horror and tell you, *"you're abusive."*

This example happened to someone I know.

I call this the ultimate energy transference. Many of us have learned this and do it without realizing it. This is when someone projects their emotions onto someone else, and the other person (because they too are masters at suppression), takes on those feelings, acts them out and then feels like they are crazy.

I invite you to consider the following:

Suppressed sadness equals depression.

Suppressed fear equals terror.

Here is a perfect quote about suppressing emotions:

"You can suppress the truth of things for only so long. Eventually its light will crack your shell and come bursting forward with uncontrollable force." ~ Amy Jalapeno

Think of it this way: Suppressing anger leads to rage, which can lead someone to abuse an animal, another human, or punch a wall. If this same person could feel whatever they felt in the moment they felt it, that emotion would flow through them in those ninety-second intervals until it had passed through them. When you allow emotional charges to build up within you, you are sitting on an emotional volcano—it will erupt at some point. Those emotions must go somewhere. I always tell clients, "Better out than in," provided it is done in a safe and healthy way where you get to release your emotions without hurting yourself or anyone else with your words or actions.

By suppressing and telling yourself you should not feel whatever you feel, you could be in the unfortunate position of having your emotions erupt so it hurts you or someone else.

So, what can you do?

How can you effectively uncover and release suppressed emotions and free the most important person in your life: you?

Tapping is by far the most effective tool I know of that allows you to do just this. As one mentor said "Show me a tool that works better, and I will use it. Until then, I use tapping." Stick with me and I will show you how to use tapping, in the most effective ways I know of to release suppressed emotions.

There Is a Way to Feel Better and Improve Your Life

It starts with feeling your emotions in all of their fullness which, as I have mentioned before and bears repeating, is something that is not promoted in our society. Therefore, it requires courage and practice because some of your emotions can feel so uncomfortable. So how do you feel your emotions while not feeling overcome by them?

Tapping is a surprising, kind of strange, yet highly effective technique that allows you to release the buildup of years of buried emotions. Once you remove the buildup you get back into alignment where you can effectively feel what you feel. When you can effectively feel what you feel (without letting them build up again), you reignite your life force—your creative energy.

When this happens, you will notice your thoughts are more positive. You will just feel better. Feeling better leads to better decisions and overall better outcomes in every area of your life, and from this place you move into an even better version of yourself and your life.

How to Make Impactful Decisions from the Heart

Having a desire for "more" or for something different than your reality is actually a good thing because this is your desire to grow. Desires are normal part of being human. It is our attachment to our desires being realized that causes most of us pain and suffering, because when our desires don't get realized, we usually end up thinking there is something wrong with us. This happens when we are attached to what we think is best, because we are actually closing ourselves off to things being realized in our lives that can be even greater than we can image.

I am not suggesting that you should be cavalier about your life and your commitments. Rather, I am suggesting that when you have a desire—an inner nudge, if you will—that is prompting you to take inspire action, you consider it thoughtfully. When you pay attention to and move with this energy you are allowing something potentially even better to come into being for you. You are allowing an expanded awareness to take the lead and amazing things can come from this. When you do this, you act out of inspiration. You create from inspiration instead of the "have to's" and "should's" and "just get it done's" that life programs us to believe are the ways it should be.

The litmus test for making decisions is—does it feel light or heavy to you? Understand you are in the best state of consciousness when you feel light, uplifted, and inspired. Things feel easier.

Now you might be asking, "Is that even possible and if so, how can I get there?

Yes, it is possible, and in the next chapter I will share an exercise to help you become more in tune with your thoughts, so you can use them to make the best decisions.

Chapter Summary

To recap: Most of us have no idea that our before picture isn't working for us, until we start to feel frustrated or stuck in a life that's not working anymore for us.

We come to know things aren't working because of the emotions that are coming up for us. In this way, our emotions can serve to really guide us. (This will be discussed more in Chapter 2.)

Real lasting change often starts from seeing what's not working in your life.

As you start to see what's not working the desire to have a new life experience that far more empowering starts with normalizing every single thought and emotion you have and understanding how beliefs that limit us get established in us.

Through this understanding, you start to notice evidence of the after picture appearing in your life.

You know this in the following ways:

Comparing yourself to others diminishes.

Negative thinking starts to be replaced with more positive thinking.

Criticizing other begins to soften.

You find you are reacting less and responding more.

Overreacting calms down.

You allow space to go into emotions and allow them to move through you.

You might even notice emotions waving through you in 90 second intervals.

You notice that you're feeling "lighter" especially if you practice interrupting negative thinking over a sixty-day period. This becomes evidence your physiology is changing.

You become more accepting and less afraid of your feelings.

You begin to recognize that your thought just fires off. You can't stop them, but you know you can interrupt them. This bring a sense of freedom from fearing your thoughts and the emotions tied to them.

All of your feelings become a normal part of being human rather than needing to be eradicated. As you're feeling more fully, you may notice that decisions get made through you, rather than by you because now you're starting to tune into your intuition more.

All this ultimately adds up to a far more liberated life.

Thoughts and Voices

Pay Attention to Your Thoughts

You have likely heard that awareness is a great first step, and it is true. When you become aware of your thoughts, this is where you can change them when needed. Here is a classic and simple but not necessarily easy exercise: pay attention to your thoughts. If you have to place Post-It Notes around your home or reminders on your phone to remind you to stop and listen to your thoughts, do it. Spend whatever amount of time that feels manageable to you and work your way up to longer periods of time. Notice your thoughts as often as you can. That having been said, I am not suggesting that you have to walk around all day paying attention to your thoughts; do so off and on throughout the day to help notice limiting thoughts, and especially pay attention when things seem to head south for you emotionally or when you are feeling triggered. To clarify, let me explain what I mean by being triggered.

I like this definition of trigger.

"Triggers are anything that remind someone of previous trauma. To be triggered is to have an intense emotional or physical reaction, such as a panic attack, after encountering a trigger."[2]

When I am triggered, I am having an emotional and physical response that hijacks my ability to remain calm. My physiology would show I have elevated cortisol levels (the stress hormone) and this moves energy away from my prefrontal cortex (the thinking, reasoning, creative part of the brain). The redirection of energy doesn't allow me access to this part of the brain.

When I am aware of this, I can tap in the moment I am triggered to help release the stress response I am having to a particular circumstance. I find this is actually the best time to tap, because it helps to release the stress response. Now instead of being hijacked emotionally and physically, I am able to calm myself and this allows me to respond rather than react. This is so valuable for stressful life events.

Years ago, my husband and I went through a rough time financially. I am not exaggerating when I say that for about a year I did not sleep through the night. I would fall asleep, but in the middle of the night I would be jarred awake by what I call my "racing thoughts."

It sucked.

I could not conjure up a positive thought. I was drowning in thoughts that stirred up fear, terror, panic, and anxiety (talk about a cesspool of dark thoughts). A series of thoughts would pop in my head one on top of the other.

"What if we end up homeless?"

"Oh my God, we have two girls, how are we going to take care of them?"

"I'm in my later 40s and I have nothing to show for it financially."

"I'm screwed."

"Why did I attract this into my life?"

Talk about debilitating.

I tried to think positive thoughts and felt incapable of it. I would say affirmations, but they never landed for me. They had the opposite effect; I felt worse because I judged myself for my inability to get into a positive frame of mind. I would lie there with these dark, racing thoughts regurgitating through my brain, and would beg for sleep to come so I could escape them.

I did not know this then, but I later researched why it seems so hard to change thoughts.

What I found coalesced into the research I found through Dr. Bruce Lipton, Lynne McTaggert, Jordan Lejuwaan, and the study conducted through the US National Library of Medicine National Institutes of Health I referenced in the last chapter.

Essentially, each emotion we experience—sadness, happiness, anger, and so on—releases its own neuropeptides that move through the body and affect our cells. When we experience a lot of anger, for example, it connects with anger receptors in the cells, changing the cells' structure. When the cells divide, if they have been exposed to lots of anger and little happiness, the new cells will be more receptive to anger, and less receptive to happiness.

Consistently negative thoughts program our very cells to be more receptive to negativity (and less receptive to positivity).

From Dr. Bruce Lipton's work if the environment affects the cells, as we release the negative emotions, we make space for positive emotions to take root again.

I did not know this back when I was caught on the hamster wheel of negative thinking, but here is what happened:

About a year into this madness, I woke up one morning and, as I got out of bed, my skin felt like it was on fire. It was so itchy that if I would have had a drill with a sanding tool on the end, I would have used it. I looked in the mirror and found that my entire body was covered in hives. I was mortified at the image looking back at me, and the thought popped into my head, *"Marti, you're literally killing yourself with your thoughts."*

It was not a judgmental thought. It felt like a compassionate voice was giving me a message I understood to be true as soon as I heard it. The next thought that came was the idea that I might find one tiny little thing to feel grateful for each day. I understood that I was incapable of just suddenly thinking positively; I had tried so often, and it had never worked.

What I know now is that I had too much momentum going with my negative thinking, and I was unconsciously programming my cells for more negative thinking (no wonder I could not conjure a positive thoughts). What I did do was suggesting to myself that I might find one tiny thing to feel a little gratitude for. I kept the bar low hoping I would find a measure of success with this, and I did.

Ninety-nine-point-nine percent of the day, my thoughts were in the toilet, but I found that one little ray of light each day—something I could feel grateful for. I am talking small moments in my day.

"The clerk at the grocery store smiled at me. I can feel grateful for this."

"That guy in that car waved me into his lane. I can feel grateful for this."

"The tea I had this morning was nice and warm going down. I can feel grateful for this."

37

Looking back, I see what I had slowly done; I had shifted my focus to look for what was appealing in my life instead of only noticing everything that was not working.

This little exercise interrupted my dark thoughts. I could not stop the dark thoughts from coming, but I could interrupt them. I did not realize that is what I was doing. I just practiced finding one thing— just one—to feel grateful for. Let me reiterate, it was a practice. Ultimately, by interrupting my negative thoughts via looking for something positive to hold on to, I was reprogramming my cells toward more positive thoughts. It is also interesting to note it was between sixty and ninety days when I started to notice I was feeling better and more positive.

From my experience, you can begin to notice a change in the way you feel if you consistently using tapping every day to create momentum. Each one of us is different, but you will/may be tapping every day for around sixty days, and then one day you notice that you are not so reactive to life events that in the past have triggered you. You notice little wins here and there. You may find that where you used to get upset when someone criticizes you, now you do not care so much. You notice you are not taking things as personally. You are more detached. The added benefit is you literally feel freer emotionally. When this happens, you draw more positive thoughts to you because you have momentum in moving toward more positive life experiences.

This is important to know: I could not stop the long practiced dark thoughts because they had too much momentum going. The practice of finding something to feel grateful for slowly helped me to shift my focus, and thus my thoughts, toward lighter, more positive thoughts. I was literally interrupting the negative momentum in tiny increments by looking for one small thing to feel some gratitude about.

Over time, it had a profound effect on me.

I was unknowingly reprogramming my cells by changing my inner environment.

Woo-hoo!

Just imagine how being aware of this can help you. I was beating myself up repeatedly for not thinking positively, and this only created more resistance in an already challenging situation. This is often a place where people give up and think, "this positive, grateful crap doesn't work." I will continue with my experience to illustrate what I mean.

Before feeling grateful for just one little thing came to me, I was attempting to leap from hellish thoughts to happy thoughts in one fell swoop, and it was not working. The negative momentum was too strong.

It could not have worked because my cells were programmed for negative thoughts, so it was way too big of a jump. I now understand more fully how positive thinking, and using it to change your life, works. You have to start small, in tiny increments. It is two steps:

Use Tapping (also known as Emotional Freedom Techniques or EFT) to deal directly with your negative thoughts. This is such a relief. You no longer have to fear your negative thoughts because now you can go into them and tap on them to release them.

Begin to slowly cultivate gratitude and appreciation. Find the little wins/the smallest things to appreciate, e.g., *"My emotions were really negative today, but at least I tapped on them."*

If you are a believer in The Law of Attraction, you will also see The Law of Attraction in a new way.

The following comes from American author, motivational speaker, corporate trainer, and entrepreneur, Jack Canfield.

"What is The Law of Attraction?

The Law of Attraction says that you will attract into your life whatever you focus on. Whatever you give your energy and attention to will come back to you." Jack Canfield

If you stay focused on the good and positive things in your life, you will automatically attract more good and positive things into your life. If you are focused upon lack and negativity, then you will attract it into your life.

Here is how it works:

Like attracts like. If you are feeling excited, enthusiastic, passionate, happy, joyful, appreciative, or abundant, then you are sending out positive energy.

But if you are feeling bored, anxious, stressed out, angry, resentful, or sad, you are sending out negative energy.

The universe, through The Law of Attraction, will respond enthusiastically to both of these vibrations. It does not decide which one is better for you, it just responds to whatever energy you are creating, and it gives you more of the same. You get back what you put out there.

Whatever you are thinking and feeling is basically your request to the universe for more of the same. Because your energy vibrations will attract energy back to you of the same frequencies, you need to make sure that you are continually sending out energy, thoughts, and feelings that resonate with what you want to be, do, and experience.

Your energy frequencies need to be in tune with what you want to attract in your life.

If joy and love are what you want to attract, then the vibrational frequencies of joy and love are what you want to create."

You do not have to believe in this law for the techniques in this book to help you. I have many clients from all walks of life who have benefited greatly from the teachings in this book without ever believing in The Law of Attraction. However, if you can suspend your rational mind, and thus judgment, and "feel" in your body if this makes even an inkling of sense to you, great. If it does not, no problem—utilize whatever does make sense to you. I encourage you to trust yourself.

If you have ever studied Law of Attraction (which is often misinterpreted; I will explain shortly), if you think good and happy thoughts, you will energetically emit a vibrational frequency—like a magnet—that will attract into your experience that which you are putting out there.

If you think repetitive thoughts like, *"That is just my luck,"* and your meaning behind it is, *"With my luck, things are not going to work out for me,"* guess what—things will not work out for you.

Then you might say something like, *"See, I told you it would not work out. This is just my luck."*

I have had this thinking myself: desperately wanting for things to change in my life and yet my true thoughts about it all was that my life was not going to change. I was programmed to think this way, and if you are reading this book, it is likely you were.

I coached with an amazing woman, Dina Proctor, who wrote the book, Madly Chasing Peace: How I Went from Hell to Happy in 9 Minutes a day. During one session together, she said, "Marti, if you'd bet money on it, this is your point of attraction." That landed for me because I immediately understood what she meant.

41

She meant that if I have already drawn a conclusion in my mind, and I am so convinced something will turn out a certain way that I would bet money on it, then I have already determined the results. By doing so, I will create the circumstances for those results to happen, good or bad. My energy is affecting the outcome.

Having been raised in a devout Catholic household, I was never exposed to anything like this. From my understanding, nothing was in my control; (nothing really is actually in our control) it was all up to the God of my understanding to bestow His good will on me if He deemed me worthy.

I went to a Catholic funeral for a dear friend, and I was reminded of this statement we were taught to say at every mass. "Lord, I am not worthy to receive, but only say the word and my soul shall be healed." I repeated this phrase for decades, literally programming myself to believe that I was unworthy. Personally, I think it is unfortunate to walk through life believing we are not worthy. As you might guess, I chose a long time ago to no longer practice the religion I was raised with. It is for you to decide what is best for you.

The Law of Attraction offered a different way of seeing things, and it made more sense. My energy, through what I focus on, creates what I am experiencing. From this viewpoint, I can create either heaven or hell in my experiences right here on planet Earth. Wow! Now, this may bump hard up against whatever you believe; it did for me when I first learned about The Law of Attraction, but when I looked back through my life and what I would experience, it was like the curtain fell away and a ray of hope got through.

Until another curtain blocked my vision, that is. Until I beat myself up for attracting bad things into my life because The Law of Attraction, when it is not understood, can be just another way to beat yourself up. Here is an example of what I mean by this: you attract a person, circumstance, or experience into your life, and you do not like it. Then you think some version of:

"Well, I attracted this into my life."

"I must not be doing this right."

"There's just something wrong with me."

Now, I ask you, does that series of thoughts make you feel better or worse?

Before I talk more about The Law of Attraction and specifically one teaching of Abraham Hicks I find very useful, *The Emotional Guidance Scale*, I want to add that in my twenties and thirties I was and still am a believer in the spiritual concepts of Divine Order, Divine Timing, Divine Selection. Something I became familiar with through a Unity Church I attended when I lived in the Chicago area. Charles and Myrtle Fillmore were the founders of Unity.

Whether you have heard of these concepts or not, whether you believe them or not, they worked well in my own life for many years.

I lost touch with these ideas for many years and old wounds took over. Tapping helped me navigate through the muck of limiting beliefs and emotionally charged events from my childhood. Within the last few years when I found myself exhausted from *"trying to think positively"* and *"trying to manifest"* I found myself exhausted and discouraged because some things desired came into being while other things I desired did not. This elevated my feelings of discouragement, even though I was tapping.

So why do somethings happen while others don't? My conclusion and I've heard many other believers in The Law of Attraction mirror the following thought, "It must be my fault."

This sucked because I went back into self-blame, much like Catholicism. It got brought home when a friend said "Marti, I think you're using The Law of Attraction to beat yourself up."

Whoa, she was right. So why don't we always manifest what we want?

I was reintroduced to Divine Order, Divine Timing and Divine Selection once again by a woman named Tosha Silver. Once again, when I was at wits end, this reintroduction came as a welcome relief.

Tosha's so beautiful answers why we do not get what we desire.

I am paraphrasing here, but she suggests:

What if when we don't manifest what we desire it's because we're being redirected to something much better. Something greater than we can image than when we're caught in our ego-based awareness. There is also the Law of Karma, meaning we come into this life with things that are designed for our soul's evolution. So sometimes that things we want, aren't in the best interest for our evolution.

What a relief! This has been so helpful in relieving the burden of self-judgment. You can learn more about Tosha and these teachings at toshasilver.com.

Now back to the aspects The Law of Attraction I find helpful.

If you listen to Law of Attraction leaders like Esther Hicks with Abraham, you will hear talk about your Emotional Guidance Scale. I have heard them repeatedly say some version of: *"If you are in despair and you want to feel joy, you cannot make that leap immediately—it is too big of an emotional leap. You have to move yourself up the emotional scale and reach for the next-best-feeling thought."*

If you are feeling despair and you can move yourself up the scale toward anger, you have moved in the right direction. This was liberating for me; it was such a relief. Add on to this how we can reprogram our cells from negative thinking to positive thinking and you can understand what you are being encouraged toward by The Law of Attraction: to slowly and steadily reach for a thought that brings you some measure of relief.

During my time of the financial crisis, when I was lying in bed night after night feeling unable to eke out a positive thought, I was in my own private hell. I was trying to feel good when I was in a pit of despair. I was trying to move myself to a feeling completely out of reach for me. From this place of despair, I was telling myself to just think positively and just get happy. It was impossible. I was judging myself harshly for not getting positive.

When I woke up that one morning and saw the hives and realized what my chronic negative thinking was doing to my health, it moved something in me. I started small and tried to find one thing throughout my entire waking day I could feel some small sense of appreciation for. I could find relief from my negative thinking. It worked because I was not trying to get happy. I was just trying to take a small step toward feeling better, and over time I did feel incrementally better, and then a little better and then a little better. This happened over a couple of months. Imagine that.

This is what gets missed in The Law of Attraction. People try positive thinking and when they do not get results, they either beat themselves up for attracting the bad stuff, or they get discouraged because they think it does not work for them.

It does work, but it is a natural step-by-step progression that comes with time.

Your Roadmap to Better Feelings

If you find yourself stuck in a certain emotional state, the Emotional Guidance Scale below can help you pull yourself up the scale to an emotion that feels a little less painful.

It is a roadmap that allows you to move yourself to a better feeling, more manageable place over time, without the pressure of having to make the leap from misery to joy.

Emotions are rated in order, from top to bottom, with what most people would agree are the better feeling emotions to the not-so-good feeling emotions.

The Emotional Guidance Scale by Abraham Hicks

Joy/Appreciation/Empowerment/Freedom/Love
Passion
Enthusiasm/Eagerness/Happiness
Positive Expectation/Belief
Optimism
Hopefulness
Contentment
Boredom
Pessimism
Frustration/Irritation/Impatience
Overwhelm
Disappointment
Doubt
Worry
Blame
Discouragement
Anger
Revenge
Hatred/Rage
Jealousy
Insecurity/Guilt/Unworthiness
Fear/Grief/Depression/Despair/Powerlessness

In a book titled "*Ask and It Is Given: Learning to Manifest Your Desires,*" authors Esther Hicks and Jerry Hicks write:

"Imagine a time in your life when you felt despair, which is #22, and you want to get to positive expectation, which is #4. If you put pressure on yourself to feel better, because someone tells you that you need to get happy, this adds more pressure, you cannot do it. You just cannot."[3]

It is important to know the voice telling you to get happy, whether it is your own or someone else's, actually promotes you to deny emotion. It is a bully. Most of us have done enough self-bullying to last us a lifetime. With that in mind, let's talk about the Noisy Companions you share your head space with.

Mastering Your Noisy Companions

Let's talk about "Parts Work" in the Internal Family Systems Model. The Center for Self-Leadership outlines the Internal Family Systems Model.

Basic Assumption of the IFS Model from Internal Family Systems

It is the nature of the mind to be subdivided into an indeterminate number of sub-personalities, or parts.

Everyone has a Self, and the Self can and should lead the individual's internal system.

The non-extreme intention of each part is something positive for the individual. There are no "bad" parts, and the goal of therapy is not to eliminate parts but instead to help them find their non-extreme roles.

As we develop, our parts develop and form a complex system of interactions among themselves; therefore, systems theory can be applied to the internal system. When the system is reorganized, parts can change rapidly.

Changes in the internal system will affect changes in the external system and vice versa. The implication of this assumption is that both the internal and external levels of system should be assessed.

You can learn more about Internal Family Systems at their website The Center for Self-leadership at this website. https://selfleadership.org.

I worked with a coach who introduced me to Internal Family Systems and the Basics Assumptions of the IFS Model mentioned and it helped me to practice separating from the different parts in myself. I am the type of person who can complicate a potato chip, so I simplified this for myself and ultimately for my clients, but my variation is based in the Internal Family Systems Method.

This method goes hand in hand for me with the following quote from Eckhart Tolle's book, *Practicing the Power of Now:*

"The beginning of freedom is the realization that you are not 'the thinker.' The moment you start watching the thinker, a higher level of consciousness becomes activated. You then begin to realize that there is a vast realm of intelligence beyond thought, that thought is only a tiny aspect of that intelligence. You also realize that all the things that truly matter—beauty, love, creativity, joy, inner peace—arise from beyond the mind. You begin to awaken."[4]

What I have found is that when you notice who is running the show within you, you can better practice a new way of seeing yourself which helps you to manage your emotional state better instead of unconsciously allowing it to run you. "You start watching the thinker," as Eckhart Tolle states.

Here is how I have simplified the Internal Family Systems Model:

I see this as having three parts of interest to us.

1) The Bully in Your Brain
2) Your Wounded Child
3) Your Healthy Adult Self

I will explain each part separately.

1) The Bully in Your Brain

Before I knew anything about this work, I learned of a part within me I used to say was the part trying to kill me. It felt this way because it was brutal. It felt like it bullied me all the time.

Even though I noticed this part, I did not see how I was using this voice to judge myself harshly. The Bully in Your Brain is that relentless part that has you riddled with self-judgment. Interestingly, most of us do not even realize how often we bully ourselves. We have become so accustomed to it we do not notice its prevalence. We have heard this voice most of the day and we have fallen asleep to it, so we do not even think about it. Noticing the Bully is critical to allowing yourself to move through emotions more readily.

I define the Bully in Your Brain this way: it is all the critical self-talk in your brain that leaves you feeling debilitated or feeling bad about yourself. When you notice that you are feeling bad about yourself, if you pay attention to the thoughts rumbling around in your brain, I think you will find you are relentlessly criticizing yourself.

The Bully sounds like these statements:

"I'll never make it."

"I'm too old."

"I'm too young."

"Who do you think you are?"

"Keep a stiff upper lip."

"I'm so pathetic."

"Just get it done it."

"I can't believe I was so stupid."

"You can't make a living being a musician."

"Do you know what small percentage of the population makes it?"

"Your best bet is to get a job with benefits. You are much safer this way."

And any variation of these lovely sentiments.

On and on ad nauseam. There are oodles of them.

As you pay attention to your thoughts, see if you notice a critical part within yourself. It intends to protect you, like an overprotective parent yelling at you not to touch a hot stove, or a guidance counselor who takes one look at your report card and tells you not to reach too high because your grades do not reflect someone who could succeed in a career such as a lawyer. They do not want you to get hurt or disappointed, but in their effort to save you from yourself, they are limiting you.

Now, this being said, I call your nagging voice the Bully because this part leaves you feeling beat up emotionally. It does not cut you any slack. It seems to have a keen sense of when to pounce. I find it parachutes in when you are feeling your most vulnerable and drops a heaping pile of limitation on you, as in the above statements.

Sometimes this critical part surges when you feel emotionally vulnerable. This voice shows judgment around your vulnerability, not an acceptance of it. When judgment is present around your vulnerability, you feel the wounds of your inner Wounded Child. The concept of a Wounded Child has been around for a long time. I like using this term here because of its clarity.

2) Your Wounded Child

You can recognize the Wounded Child whenever you have a high emotional charge, meaning when you are deep in the throes of emotion that seems out of proportion to the situation. This is an indicator that your Wounded Child is running your show. When you check in, you feel as powerless as you did when you were a child. This indicates your Wounded Child has been activated.

One day a therapist I worked with said, *"Your inner kid is activated."* That simple statement did wonders for me. In that moment, I understood this was a part of me, but it was not all of who I am. Before that, I so identified with this wounded part of me I never separated myself from it.

I have come to recognize in myself and within clients that the Wounded Child gets activated and the Bully jumps in with fear mongering. The Bully pounds the Wounded Child to dust with all kinds of debilitating statements. It creates a vicious cycle.

Using my earlier example of the stressful financial time when I could not sleep through the night, the conversation between parts goes something like:

I would wake up feeling terrified, which meant my Wounded Child was activated. I would lay in terror trying to feel better and then my Bully would start its barrage. "You're a loser. How could you have let this happen? What the hell is wrong with you? Look at all the people on the planet your age who are so much better off than you are."

52

(I have never been privy to anyone else's financial statement, so in hindsight, I understand how ludicrous this last statement was. This kind of bullying self-talk is debilitating.)

In the moment, The Bully had my Wounded Child reeling in terror of being homeless and not surviving. The more my Wounded Child panicked, the more the Bully would relentlessly feed her debilitating thoughts, and the more she would panic. A vicious cycle.

It is like an older child bullying a younger child, and it does not stop until an adult steps in. This brings us to the third part.

3) Your Healthy Adult Self

When we are born, we have two parts: our Spiritual Self (Higher Self) and our Human Self. These two parts are intertwined and work together. Your Higher Self collaborates with your Human Self and delivers information to it that is always positive. It does this even when we are children.

As we grow past childhood, I call the Human Self the Healthy Adult Self. This receives guidance from the Higher Self and understands what is needed.

The information that your Spiritual Self delivers to your Healthy Adult Self comes more as a feeling of knowing, a sense of understanding not expressed in words. Your Healthy Adult Self integrates this in words that the other parts of you can hear, whether they can grasp them yet or not. The Healthy Adult Self thus understands how to soothe both the Bully and the Wounded Child. Your Healthy Adult Self can then implement more empowering behaviors.

Remember that you were born with this Human Self, or Healthy Adult Self. More often than not we learn to believe that things are missing from us and that we have to bring into our being what is missing. This could not be further from the truth. Instead, we have to remove the negative emotional undertow we adopted over years of programming so we can have access to our true nature. As we clear out our baggage, we uncover and reconnect with our inner wisdom, guidance, and support.

Below are three effective steps to assist this Healthy Adult Self to take the lead in your life.

Three Step Process to Change Who is Running Your Show

1) Awareness

You notice you are triggered. You are having a strong emotional charge, which tells you that your Wounded Child has been activated. An inner battle ensues between your Wounded Child and the Bully in Your Brain. Your Wounded Child is in reaction mode, and then your Bully comes in with all the things you "should" or "shouldn't" be doing. Awareness alone is the first way to interrupt the pattern.

2) Interrupt with a question

Once you are aware your child is activated (again, you know this because of the strong emotion that seems out of proportion to the situation), ask yourself this question: How old do I feel right now? More often than not, an age will come to mind. Two things happen when you do this:

You create a pattern interrupt because you interrupted the train of emotion with a question.

You put your adult self back in charge. Who is asking this question? It is your adult self.

3) Soothe

Now that you have identified how old you feel, or at least that your Wounded Child is activated along with the Bully, you can soothe these parts with EFT, also known as Tapping, which I will discuss in Chapter 5.

Three Step Process Examples

In my above example, following these steps to change who is running my show might play out like this:

I wake up with a feeling of panic. I am emotionally distraught, indicating my Wounded Child has been activated and is running my show. I am experiencing this high emotional charge. My Wounded Child is reeling in terror. Now my Bully gets activated and parachutes in with statements like the following.

"You need to think positive thoughts."

"Get over it already."

"Pull it together."

Step 1: Awareness.
Wow! My kid is really activated. She is in terror.

Step 2: Interrupt with a question.
How old do I feel right now? Six comes to mind.

Step 3: Soothe.
I would tap here and speak my truth out loud, saying something like the following while tapping:

"My six-year-old self is really in fear right now. She does not feel safe. She is waiting for the worst to happen. She is overwhelmed. She is too young to handle what is going on here. She cannot see a way out. When she is running my show, my problem-solving ability is out the freaking window. I have an inner six-year-old who is trying to make grown-up decisions she is not capable of making. No wonder she is freaking out. I want to let her know that I have got this. I may not know the answer yet, but I am confident the answer will come from a calmer mind."

"Boy, my inner Bully is really activated right now as well. It really has a grip on my little kid, and that is not helping. I am going to let this Bully know that I am taking over now. I have got this and, just like a loving parent, I am going to calm all parts down. No one is getting left behind here. We're all on this journey together, but I'm in charge now, and I'm running this show."

For anyone who might be thinking, Whiskey, Tango, Foxtrot? (WTF?) What is she talking about? This sounds crazy! I know how you feel.

I say this because when I first got introduced to Parts Work, I resembled the eyeball-rolling emoji on iPhones. I was the one thinking, "This is crazy. This is ridiculous."

But I have learned to suspend my eyeball-rolling judgment and try out new techniques to see how they work. After I have tried it, if I still want to, I can roll my eyes and then move on to something else. Not every idea or technique lands for everyone. This is not one size fits all. This is about you learning to trust yourself while you investigate and explore and see what feels best to you. This said, I recommend you try whatever idea or technique presents itself to you before deciding to take it or leave it.

When I gave tapping a chance, it blew me away how this process helped me separate myself from my Wounded Child when I noticed myself overreacting. It also helped me notice when my Bully got activated and I was kicking the shit out of myself.

My clients tell me how helpful this has been. They judge themselves less and accept themselves more. They find they stop saying things to themselves like, "I'm just a mess," which now gets replaced with, "Oh wow, my kid is activated right now."

Who can't use more self-acceptance?

This 3-step process to change who's running your show helps with practicing what Eckhart Tolle describes as, "Becoming the observer of your thoughts."

Once you learn to identify when these parts of you are activated, you take your power back. Instead of your highly charged emotions running you unconsciously, you notice them, and notice the part driving them. This simple act of noticing when your Wounded Child and/or the Bully in Your Brain are active creates a separation between you and them. This separation is a helpful step toward lasting change.

I am not suggesting that you walk around all day constantly paying attention to who is running your show, but when you set the intention to bring your unconscious into your conscious awareness, you will notice when you are not feeling good emotionally. You will notice when you have an over-the-top strong emotional charge and will then recognize that the Bully and the Child are at battle, and therefore running your show. From there you can follow my 3-step process to change who is running your show.

The more you notice them, the more you can interrupt these patterns, and the more you interrupt these patterns, the more you will find that your Healthy Adult Self runs your show more often than not.

When your Healthy Adult Self runs the show, you will notice big changes with your behavior when you are triggered. At first, you might notice that you are not reacting in the same way. You might even notice that things that used to trigger you do not seem to do so in the same way. You will be calmer than you were before. You will also likely notice you feel better in general. Often, people say they feel lighter. "Lighter" is a common word used to describe how these changes feel.

If you are someone who often goes into battle mode with others, you will find you catch yourself much more quickly. You might even pull out of a potential argument and walk away because you have become more discerning about what battles to fight.

If you are someone who keeps your mouth shut when you want to say things, you may notice you speak up for yourself more, even if your voice is shaking while you are doing so. This will continue to get easier for you.

The changes can happen gradually as you start to be kinder to yourself because you are not constantly identifying with your Wounded Child or your Bully. It is liberating, and an added benefit is that you will be well on your way to setting the stage to releasing what has been blocking you from allowing guidance and direction that can help you take inspired action on the way to experience a life you love.

Chapter Summary

For quick reference and review, here, I summarize the Change Who is Running Your Show Process:

The Bully in Your Brain—whenever you notice a punitive, critical voice speaking to yourself, this is the Bully.

Your Wounded Child—whenever you notice a high emotional charge seems out of proportion to the situation, it indicates that your Wounded Child is activated and is running the show.

Your Healthy Adult Self—this is your Human Self, or your emotionally intelligent self. It is the part of you that thoughtfully considers all of your options before responding and has the self-confidence to handle whatever situation you are facing with emotional intelligence. If you believe in a power greater than yourself, this works in cooperation with your Higher Self.

On Feeling Fully

What Does It Mean to Feel Fully?

What does it mean to feel fully? Many people, when they hear this term, answer this way.

"No, thanks, I will pass. What's good about that?"

But what if I told you the significant upside of feeling fully was more freedom for you? Feeling fully means giving yourself emotional freedom, which creates emotional intelligence. Allowing yourself to release stuck emotions and feel fully activates your creative energy.

Why?

Because a host of stuck emotions no longer blocks you from accessing your intuitive, creative self. Your creative self is the very thing that allows you to feel inspired and then act from this inspiration.

Feeling fully is all about allowing emotions to move through you unencumbered and, when you do this, the feelings do not stay stuck. They move through you as intended.

When not bogged down with stuck emotions, you free up your energy, and you will notice you can be more positive. When you are more positive, you attract better circumstances, people, and events in your life.

Most of us learned a long time ago to fear painful emotions. They are the grim reaper, always looming, waiting to pounce and debilitate you.

You learned you are your emotions.

If you feel out of sorts and confused, you think things like, *"I am just a mess,"* and you believe you are just a mess and nothing else. You become the emotion instead of just feeling the emotion. This thinking shuts you down.

When bogged down with emotional baggage, solutions to challenges feel out of reach. I call this *"circling the drain emotionally."* You are waiting for the worst to happen and getting sucked down into a black hole full of stuck emotions.

But when you feel fully, and you feel through the emotions, you catch yourself. You are not your emotional state. Your emotions are just something you are experiencing. You see your emotions as indicators of where you are instead of your emotions running you.

When your emotions are not running you, you have the choice and the ability to respond instead of reacting. You are calmer because supercharged emotions no longer overwhelm you, and because you are feeling your emotions fully as they come and allowing them to dissipate.

As you go through this process, you realize you will not die from feeling fully. You will not go crazy and not be able to handle your emotions. You might find you enjoy feeling fully, as it is incredible. You have more depth in your life experiences, all helping to create a vibrant, abundant life.

Sound too good to be true? Too simple, maybe? Hang in with me, and you will get to experience what I'm telling you. But first, let's talk about why we do not feel fully.

Why Don't You Feel Fully?

Fortunately, it is not your fault. Feeling fully is not something we support by default. Centuries of programming block our embracing feelings. What does this mean? It means they programmed you growing up to reject your emotions—some more than others. They trained you not to trust yourself. How does this rejection of your emotions begin?

From the time we are babies, our parents often scoop us up and tell us not to cry, and this continues through the rest of our lives. In this way, parents reject their children's big emotions and insist they stop them or suppress them rather than feeling them. Imagine how the world might shift if, instead of telling our children, "Stop crying!" and "Go to your room until you calm down," a new generation of parents said, "It is okay to feel sad. I am here for you. I'll help you through this big emotion."

Our childhood programming of not trusting ourselves begins in other, less straightforward ways. Below are several examples.

A little boy has just finished a snack, and he says to his mom, "Mom, I'm still hungry." His mom looks at him and replies, "You cannot be hungry. You just ate." The little boy feels confused. His stomach is growling, which tells him he is still hungry, but his mother (who he believes knows best), is telling him he cannot be hungry. Self-doubt gets installed, and he learns he cannot trust what he feels.

A little girl is sitting on the couch in her family's living room, shivering. She tells her dad she is cold, to which he looks at her and says, "You cannot be cold. The temperature is 70 degrees." Her body tells her she is cold, but her father must know best, so she doubts her reality and thus doubts herself.

As this denial of a child's experience by an authority figure is repeated, the child feels self-doubt and learns not to trust what he or she is feeling. When children do not trust their feelings, they reject and even deny them. When they reject their feelings, they avoid them. Avoiding their feelings causes them to rely on their intellect for answers.

They avoid feeling, and they learn to think about their feelings instead of feeling their feelings. What this means is they intellectualize, use their rational mind when talking about feelings, therefore they are not tuned into the feelings. It is a survival tactic.

As a child, I became masterful at zipping up into my head when emotions surfaced. I would intellectualize my feelings, which goes back to thinking about my feelings instead of feeling them. As an example, when I received the phone call that my mother died, the voice on the other end asked me if I was driving. I said, "Yes, I'm driving, but I know what that means."

I knew they would say my mother was dead. I became very rational about knowing she was dead, but before I allowed myself to feel fully, I looked for a place to pull my car over. I stayed very rational, and then once I pulled over, I said, "She's dead, isn't she?" All rational, no emotional connection until I heard the words, "Yes, she's dead."

Ironically, once I heard those words, I burst into tears, and the very rational voice on the other end said: "Martha, you're not going to do your mother any good like this."

It was so enlightening. It was something I heard all the time as a child. Now, I was in a 44-year-old body, but at the moment, my 6-year-old self was activated. It stopped my emotional experience about my mother dying in its tracks. I was told once again; my feelings are not okay. It shocked me out of my grief for a moment. Fortunately, I had a voice now, I replied, "I don't think my mother cares about that now, she's dead."

This woman had learned, like most of us, to forbid emotions. In her discomfort, she learned to cut people off when they felt fully. She is a product of our culture.

When I hung up with her, I made the phone calls to my sisters, business-like, and matter of fact. Yet on the drive to my hometown, I allowed myself a fuller expression of my grief. I took a journey through my emotional landscape and the entire experience. I was more conscious of allowing myself my feelings, even in the face of others around me being uncomfortable with emotions.

Here is a more severe example of why a child may not grow up to feel his emotions fully.

A little boy is sitting at the family dinner table. He is chatting away about his T-ball game and how he hit a home run. In this animated state where he feels good about himself, he accidentally knocks his glass of milk over, and it makes a mess. His father cracks the boy across the head and yells at him, calling him an idiot or a klutz or stupid. The boy not only reels from the physical abuse, but he also sinks into a pit of emotional hurt.

Here is one possible download this boy could learn: It is not safe to be noticed or shine.

It works like this: in the height of his excitement, he is feeling good about himself—he is shining. He is letting his family know that he is proud of himself. He is reliving how good it felt to hit the home run, and he is engaged in his feelings of excitement about what happened and about himself.

When his father hits him, it shocks the boy out of his excited state into a fearful state. He is feeling physical pain, and then he is taking in the derogatory words his father has said to him. He was in a peak emotional state, followed by a deep emotional low. This can create a set-up in the brain that tells the boy it is dangerous to feel too good.

From this experience, he is likely to learn that mistakes are bad, stupid, and it is much better to fly under the radar. It is better to be invisible because if he gets noticed, he might suffer physical hurt and ridicule.

To keep safe, he will do whatever he can to not be seen and to not get noticed and to not shine. Unconsciously, he makes a vow not to be seen or to shine because it is not safe. Going forward, he lives his life from this unconscious belief that got installed in the experience.

This scenario can be the event that will keep this same boy from succeeding later in life in a career that requires public speaking or where he needs to be visible. When he is in the spotlight, this past event with such painful feelings attached can trigger the unconscious vow he made to himself when he was just a boy.

This experience might sabotage his chance for success because of the fear of public humiliation that started in childhood.

Here is another example.

A father is sitting next to his eight-year-old son on a nighttime flight to New York. It fills the little boy with excitement. His first time flying, and he expresses his excitement to his father as he looks out the window at all the lights sparkling. He is in awe of the entire experience and chatting up a storm about it. His father lets out a sigh and says to him, "We will be stuck in these same seats, on this same flight, for the next four hours looking at this same scene, so nothing is exciting about it."

The boy's face fell. The wind got knocked out of his little enthusiastic sails for a moment.

Now, this little guy still had resilience in him, so it did not take him more than about 5 minutes to recover and talk again, but he did not sound as enthusiastic as he had before.

The more this happens to this boy, the more he is likely to close the lid on his enthusiasm. He will learn to suppress his emotions so as not to rock the boat in his tribe. His tribe is his family of origin and with who he spends the most time.

This boy's father may have been tired and was not looking forward to the four-hour overnight flight, and in his frustration, he said what he said to his son. All parents have done this. When parents say what seems like minor things often enough, it can have a significant impact.

Now, had the father learned to go back to his son and own what he would say, it would have helped. It could have sounded something like this:

"Hey, son, I'm sorry for what I said. I am just really tired and not looking forward to this four-hour overnight flight. I would rather we were home and sleeping in our beds. I know this is your first flight, and it is a new experience for you. That is exciting. So why don't you tell me all the things you find exciting about this?"

This statement would have gone a long way to help the boy rekindle his enthusiasm and feel good about the experience. This boy's father experienced similar events in his own life, and he is passing down what he has learned, without being conscious of it.

Are Your Parents to Blame?

We could go back to Adam and Eve or the Caveman era to figure out where all this nonsense started. But the bottom line is when parents (or caregivers) learned to suppress their emotions—to avoid either physical or emotional pain or both— they did not learn how to support their children in feeling whatever the children feel.

It is also likely they did not learn how to actualize their dreams and, therefore, could not teach their children how to realize theirs.

If, however, parents are working on their emotional challenges, the likelihood they can support their children is much improved.

If your parents are the former and undermine you more than support you, it does not mean you cannot live a vibrant, happy, emotionally healthy, and fulfilling life or a life where you take inspired actions. That is what this book is about: how to create emotional intelligence for yourself, take inspired action (that doesn't feel like hard work) toward a life you find inspiring and fulfilling, and unique to you.

Over time, through releasing a lot of my limiting beliefs, I understood the ability to express healthy emotions was scarce when my parents were growing up. Until I learned how to release my emotional baggage, I felt victimized and was too pissed off at my parents to be understanding. Now I have genuine compassion and empathy for them.

I am not saying you should just jump to understanding and compassion and forgiveness.

If you've ever lamented about the mistreatment you feel you've suffered at the hands of any parents or caregivers; you may have experienced well-meaning people saying to you, "Your parents did the best they could."

Did you waver between anger and guilt at this statement? Statements like this are just another way your feelings get negated, and you stuff down more of your emotions, which only creates more suppressed anger which becomes rage or depression,

I love what one mentor, Emotional Freedom Techniques (EFT) Master Carol Look, said about this.

"My parents did the best they could, but it sucked for me."

Her words resonated with me, summing up how I felt. I had suppressed many of my feelings for a long time, so it was a relief to hear this.

How to Tell If You Suffer from Inner Rage (and What to Do About It)

I developed an eating disorder in my teens that lasted through my early thirties. Once I joined a 12-step program and freed myself from the eating disorder, I was astonished and afraid of the rage that surfaced in me.

One day while driving down the highway when I lived in Chicago, someone cut me off. The rage just exploded from within me. Fortunately, I did not engage in a confrontation. Unfortunately, I took it out on myself. I banged on the steering wheel and screamed.

I screamed with all I had in me.

Had anyone seen me, it would have embarrassed me. The rage became a physical force in me, and I had to dispel it. It needed an outlet.

I pulled over onto the shoulder of the road and continued screaming and hitting the steering wheel until I was exhausted. Then I sobbed. The kind of sobbing leaving you red-faced and puffy and blowing through an entire box of tissue. That level of sobbing.

I felt confused and inadequate because I could not believe I had the capacity for this rage. I thought there was something wrong with me.

Great! More to feel wrong about.

Looking back, part of me understood I needed to release all that rage, so whenever I would feel this way, I took a baseball bat to my mattress. I remember getting home from work one day. My then-husband looked at me and knew I was in a state of extreme anger. I give him a lot of credit because he just let me go and did not say a thing.

I went upstairs, took the bat from under the bed, and pounded on the mattress. It helped, but I hurt my neck on more than one occasion. I hurt myself more.

Often rage needs physical release, but I recommend you find a way that does not hurt you. Use something light to hit your pillow like a tennis racket, or kick at an empty cardboard box, or, better yet, a vigorous walk.

I now understand, at twenty-six, that when the rage exploded out of me, it was because of years of suppressing my emotions. Through this suppression, I had a buildup of a lot of intense emotion, in particular, rage.

Growing up, I saw a lot of my father's rage-filled fits. His rage was because of massive emotional suppression, caused by what he had gone through as a child, and later the Post Traumatic Stress Disorder (PTSD) he suffered after serving in two wars. It made sense that my go-to emotion became anger once I uncovered it. All the years of suppressed anger had turned into a rage once I allowed myself a fuller expression of what I felt.

If our ancestors had learned a healthy outlet for their emotions, most of us would have had a unique life experience with our emotions and feeling them. I believe most of us suppress emotions—an ocean of emotion in the pressure cooker of our body. The more we suppress, the more emotions build up inside of us, and the higher the potential for the emotional explosion.

With a pressure cooker, if you took the lid off without releasing the built-up pressure, it would explode, and you might suffer an injury or even be killed.

I believe it is the same for humans on an emotional level.

If you stop using the things helping you to suppress your emotions, i.e., food, alcohol, drugs, gambling, etc., and you do not have tools to assist you in handling your emotions, you might have an emotional explosion. Let me add, at some point, the things you do to suppress feelings stop working, so you end up with emotional outbursts either way.

If, however, you have the right tools and release your emotional buildup, your need for food, alcohol, drugs, gambling, etc., will diminish. You will find you release your emotions naturally, with a lot more ease, and without so much struggle. When I quit using food as my suppression tool—cold-turkey without an adequate replacement—it was confusing and painful.

With the understanding I have now, I work with clients to release built-up emotions foremost, and then their need for whatever they are using for suppression diminishes and seems to change on its own.

How to Stop Judging Yourself So Harshly

Here is my rule of thumb for behaviors for which we judge ourselves:

Anytime you do something that debilitates you (or harms you), and you try to stop it without lasting success, remember this: you have a strong internal—most likely

71

unconscious—reason for this. Conversely, anytime you are not practicing behaviors you understand would be beneficial, but you still do not practice these behaviors, it's the same thing in reverse. Either way, you are unconsciously trying to protect yourself.

Here is the kicker: it is always self-protection. Always! I find this advice helps clients to be just a little less judgmental of themselves.

Once you can uncover and release this internal programming driving this need to protect yourself, you will find you can move toward the things you desire without sabotaging your efforts. And, you realize you can stay safe as you move forward.

In my case, I learned it was not safe to shine and get attention. It is interesting that almost every time I got a promotion or wanted to do something fun for me, I would sabotage myself.

Just after graduating from college, one of my best friends and I drove out to Colorado to see about getting jobs at a resort in Vail. We got to Vail, and I met with the human resources director at one resort and got the job on the spot. He told me about housing and when I would need to be there to start work for the winter session. My friend and I drove back, excited that we had secured jobs.

When I got back home, an overwhelming sense of the need to be responsible overtook me. I got a promotion at my current job, and I had it in my head that having graduated from college, I could no longer be footloose and fancy-free.

Now that I had a college degree and a recent promotion, working at a ski resort for the winter became unacceptable.

My fears kicked in along with my coping mechanism—the eating disorder. I told myself there was no way I could go work at the ski resort with this condition flaring up. I never called my friend about my decision. She was waiting for me to call her and say, "Let's hit the road jack," but that call never came.

She called me one day.

"Well, I guess you are not going. It would have been nice to know."

I broke down on the phone and told her what was going on for me. Although she was disappointed, she was also very compassionate. I felt terrible when I hung up and, later, went to my sister and told her I needed help. I hospitalized myself to deal with the eating disorder, which helped me address the underlying emotions causing it.

Looking back, I was checking out of life because it felt too scary. I realize now, though I felt like I had to be responsible, I was also in conflict with handling the promotion. I feared them expecting too much of me, and I could not just have fun anymore, so the answer was to do neither.

The eating disorder flaring up was the excuse I needed to take a time out from the fear running through me.

What I know now is I was bumping up big time against several limiting beliefs in conflict with my desires. For example:

"I need to be responsible." (Limiting Belief) vs. "I'm not ready to be this responsible." (Desire)

"I need to be a grown-up now" (Limiting Belief) vs. "I want to have fun before I settle in." (Desire)

My desires conflicted with the limiting beliefs I had learned. When a desire competes with whatever limiting beliefs you have learned, and you do not have a robust, useful tool to deal with this internal rivalry, you sabotage yourself, just like I did.

To create positive, lasting change, feeling fully is a crucial step.

What Are the Results of Feeling Fully?

When you feel fully, you allow yourself to experience your fantastic palette of emotions. Learning to feel fully leads you back to trusting yourself. As you learn to embrace the messages coming to you from your feelings, you discover who you are. As you learn to understand your feelings and what they are telling you, you get in touch with your preferences.

They might surprise you.

You may find your beliefs about how things should be change—sometimes dramatically. Many of us have learned what to think and, thus, what to feel. But, as you pay attention to your emotional landscape, you see your preferences. They may be quite different in the best way. Things you learned to believe may no longer feel like a fit for you.

You may realize the work you are doing, for example, is not something you would have chosen if left to your own devices.

Maybe when you were younger, you wanted to be a stand-up comedian. Maybe one, or both, of your parents deterred you from such a thing because the percentage of people that make it in stand-up comedy is small, and they did not want you to get your hopes up.

So, you learned to put a lid on your enthusiasm about becoming a comedian. The excitement you had about this potential career went dormant. Instead of pursuing your dream, you do "the right thing" or "what they expect of you" by getting a business degree and landing a corporate job... like most people.

Now that you are uncovering the limiting beliefs and releasing them, you feel excited about the possibilities of your life. Using the comedian example above, you might sign up for a class, or get a mentor to help you rekindle your interest and excitement for comedy. Taking a chance on seeing where it takes you, no matter how old you are or how "unrealistic" this new dream might seem.

If you believe you are too old, here is a real-life example:

Peg Phillips has lived through Pearl Harbor, polio, peritonitis, a ruptured aorta, several broken bones, and the death of two children. That is a profound list of things for someone to live through.

When she was four years old, she knew she wanted to act. She waited 60+ years to see her dream become a reality. She did not work professionally until her late 60s, and at seventy-two, she originated the role of Ruth-Anne Miller on the CBS-TV series Northern Exposure. In 1993, she received a nomination for the Primetime Emmy Award for Outstanding Supporting Actress in a Drama Series. The show ran for five seasons.

I have always loved Peg Phillips's story. Before she realized her dream of acting, she took many detours in life. She married twice, raised four children, and worked as both a bookkeeper and an accountant. It was not until she moved back to the Seattle area in 1980 that she enrolled in drama school. She was in her mid-60s when she took acting classes and in her late 60s when they cast her as Ruth-Anne. She rekindled her zest and passion for acting that started when she was four years old.

If she decided she was too old, or it was too late, she would never have realized her dream. It could happen to you also when you get back in touch with what you feel is right for your life, and you do that by feeling fully.

Some great questions to ask yourself are:

"What do I feel?"

"What do I desire?"

"If there weren't any limitations of any kind for me, what would I do with my life?"

"If I felt inspired, what next step might I take?"

Can Feeling Fully Help to Heal Physical Ailments?

I have had the wonderful fortune of studying psychosomatics with an amazing woman from Calgary, Canada, Carole Maureen Friesen. Now I do workshops with another woman I met through Carole, named Christy Foster from Salt Lake City who teaches all about the body/mind connection here in the United States. You may wonder, what is psychosomatics?

According to Merriam-Webster:

"... of, relating to, concerned with, or involving both mind and body, the psychosomatic nature of man," — Herbert Ratner

"...of, relating to, involving, or concerned with bodily symptoms caused by mental or emotional disturbance."

Our bodies hold our emotions, and when we have spent years suppressing emotions, these stifled feelings can show up in our bodies as a disease. This physical manifestation can be anything from a dull headache to something much more severe, like a brain tumor. If we allow ourselves to feel fully by targeting an emotion, symptom, event, or limiting belief, the results can be amazing.

The most startling example of how feeling fully can change someone's health comes from a client of mine. This experience deepened my belief in body/mind connection and the importance of feeling fully.

When Mary and I worked together, they had diagnosed Mary with a benign, inoperable brain tumor.

One of her doctors ran a blood test that measured the hormones related to the tumor. She was told her hormone levels were elevated, indicating possible tumor growth. Her prognosis was not good; Mary was staring death in the face. Her doctor recommended that she try tapping. He tapped on himself and found it to be effective. She had tried many modalities, so what was one more?

We worked on past events in Mary's life. These events created a lot of built-up emotions within her. After six weeks of doing one session a week and plenty of rant tapping (which I will explain later), Mary went back to her doctor for a retest, and her hormone levels were normal. He asked her what she had been doing, and she told him she'd taken his advice to use EFTs (aka tapping).

After getting her blood work retested, Mary went to her neurosurgeons for a brain scan. They told her that her tumor had shrunk to half of what it had been, confounded at her results. They could not explain them.

During our next session, when Mary informed me of what had happened, I was astonished. I felt a wave of happiness. She attributed this massive shift to releasing suppressed emotions from past events. She said tapping was the only new thing introduced into her life.

It amazed me.

Mary's desire to live was an essential part of the shift she experienced in her health.

I also want to clarify I am not making a medical claim. I only hope to relate the possible interconnectedness of our bodies and minds, and thus emotions

Mary had significant changes not only in her physical world, but she also felt emotionally lighter and freer. When she recalled past events that once held an oppressive, heavy feeling for her, she noticed these seemed like impassive stories now. They had happened, and it was unfortunate, but the emotional charge and entanglement Mary experienced with them was no longer there. She could recall these events and feel neutral about them.

Other Potential Results from Feeling Fully

Mary also saw her business grow and enjoyed better relationships because she was showing up for herself differently. She felt more empowered, and people that had once intimidated her no longer did. They behaved differently with her.

One person, in particular, whom she'd had a past adversarial relationship, someone who intimidated her, was now asking her permission to show up for an event she was hosting. She was astonished at how this person had done a complete turnaround from before. She attributes this to having released all the emotions around their adversarial relationship.

The power lies within you. Mary's experience is an example of how powerful tapping is when people have a powerful desire to change their lives. A person's inner passion, and their firm conviction to make a change, are the most important factors I see within people who make positive changes.

We may not see how to change, yet when we set a clear intention to change, we need not know the details of how it happens. Somehow, the act of mentally and emotionally tuning in to the willingness to change creates the space for the "how to change" to show up.

Once you address the underlying emotions, not only will you find your thoughts healthier and more positive, you will notice your behaviors follow.

It can be an enormous relief when you realize the reason your health, relationships, career, and finances are not where you want them to be is not because you are defective, and something is wrong with you. It is because you learned to suppress emotions and adopted limiting beliefs that have been hard-wired within you.

Why It Is Crucial for Parents to Meet Their Children's Emotional Needs

Years ago, while struggling with my less-than-effective parenting style, I read a brilliant parenting book called Parenting with Love and Logic by Foster Kline, M.D., and Jim Fay. One of my most significant takeaways was that children's needs are best met by parents who fulfill their own needs.

Children watch what you do more than anything you say. They will model your behavior.

When you encourage children to feel what they feel, you make emotions acceptable. When you also show your children practical ways to work with their feelings, you help them create more good in their lives. Helping them to create possibilities for themselves and foster a more positive human who will affect the world in a positive way.

You do this by starting with yourself. When you work to resolve your issues, you play a role in molding the future of this planet by helping to shape amazing people to bring incredible ideas and inspirations into the world.

How Feeling Fully Can Impact Your Intimate Relationships

Let's look at how feeling fully can help in your intimate relationships.

If things have not been going well with your partner and you are the person who processes through talking, you will call a friend, or two, or three, and speak to them about your challenges.

For a while, your friends want to comfort you and validate your feelings. If, however, you keep calling them about the same issues and nothing changes, they may develop an unfavorable opinion of your significant other. This happens because most of us do not call our friends when things are going well; we do not feel the need. Things are going well, so we just enjoy it.

How often do you call your friends when your partner does something great? I am guessing it is not as often as when struggling with something. Most of us seem wired to do this. It takes practice to pay attention and take in the good someone does for us.

Imagine if you practiced calling your friends when your partner did good things that involved you. Imagine if you had another way to allow yourself to feel all the emotions you experience when your partner's behavior is less than desirable. Imagine if you could resolve the challenging issues without involving your friends all the time.

I am not suggesting for one minute this is easy. With our intimate relationships, most of us have been hard-wired to notice the shit show instead of the hit show. This is a by-product of having to suppress our feelings. Because we have not learned effective ways of dealing with upsets and resolving them in a way we feel good about, the upsets build up.

If you practice paying attention to what is right in your life, noticing the hit show can take more precedence for you. What needs to come first, however, is the ability to release suppressed emotions in a safe and healthy manner.

As you learn to release suppressed emotions, you benefit by noticing more of the hit show experiences because you have cleared the muck blocking you from seeing the good.

I remember a splendid example in my life. My husband told me something he had done that triggered my anger. I paid close attention to how angry I was feeling, and I expressed to him how angry I felt about the situation. I owned my rage instead of blaming him for it. I was feeling it and expressing it.

At that moment, he allowed the space for me to feel it. I think it helped I was not blaming him. He did not parachute in and try to fix it. He did not feel the need to get defensive because I was staying present with my feelings.

What is interesting is that, within ninety seconds, this wave of anger rolling through me passed and, even more interesting, I let it go.

The rest of that day, we had an enjoyable time together. I saw the wonderful things—the hit show.

The funny thing is, I could not tell you what he said now. I view this as a good thing because this means I did not hide it in my file drawer of past offenses, building up more suppressed emotions.

For me, this was a splendid example of how an emotion can move through your being if you allow it just to be what it is. It also showed the benefit of allowing emotion to move through you. It helped that my husband was in the space to recognize it as well because it let me own my feelings, and as a result, see how quickly an unencumbered emotion moves through me.

Had he gotten defensive, or tried to fix anything, or tried to get me not to feel the way I did, I can tell you my anger would have elevated just as fast. The space was available for him to be present and not defensive because I did not blame him. Not blaming someone when they are doing or sharing something is another benefit of dealing with your emotions.

I believe we can train ourselves to allow for all our feelings. Whether or not someone else can give us space, it helps when you are first getting acquainted with your emotional landscape to have experiences like this. These supported experiences often show the emotional freedom that is possible.

When you learn to free yourself from making yourself wrong for feeling whatever you feel, you honor yourself and your emotions. This creates the roadway to emotional freedom for yourself and tuning into your life force.

Feeling fully is the key to freeing up your life force so you can learn how to lead a more fulfilling and inspired life. When you have less static in your life, you get a clearer signal from within what steps to take to move forward, and you can better access your creativity.

Feeling fully is all about allowing your emotions to move through you. The more you allow your emotions to move through you, the better you can feel more fully in the moment. Tapping is an incredible tool to help you with this. Embracing all your emotions becomes more comfortable over time, especially when you use tapping as a tool.

There are many more benefits to feeling fully.

You liberate yourself from your past.

You become less self-judging and more self-accepting.

You trust yourself.

You respect and value and love yourself.

You plain feel more joy in your life.

Does that sound like something you would like to experience?

If so, it is critical to learn to use your emotions as guidance along your path. You do this by embracing your emotions instead of rejecting them. You rewrite how you view your emotions. Instead of them being something terrible you should avoid, they become your roadmap to emotional freedom.

And it starts with examining and unlearning how you make your emotions wrong or forbidden. In the next chapter, we will examine what I call forbidden emotions.

Chapter Summary

Learning to feel fully is a lifelong process. The more you practice how to allow yourself to embrace all of your emotions, the better you'll get at it and the freer you'll feel.

The upside of this practice is that you'll release the harsh self-judgment you've accumulated over your lifetime. The liberation of feeling fully can show up in feeling calmer emotionally. Less reactive and freer mentally, you can thus access the creative part of your brain—the prefrontal cortex—and be healthier because you've reduced cortisol levels, the stress hormone, that can flood your body.

You might find you open up to a great sense of being guided and directed by your intuition. This allows life to unfold with more ease and synchronicity.

Forbidden Emotions

What Are Forbidden Emotions?

We have learned there are good and bad, right, and wrong emotions.

Any time you tell yourself you should not be feeling whatever you are feeling, you are facing a Forbidden Emotion.

You subconsciously, or consciously, reject these emotions and therefore feel you should resist or get over them quickly.

This rejection creates more resistance, which elevates both the frequency and intensity with which you feel the Forbidden Emotions. Feelings do not just disappear into thin air if you do not feel them fully; they get buried inside of you, and they have a way of coming out when you least expect it. Often at an inopportune time.

Physical Signs of Forbidden Emotions

Physical cues can determine if you are experiencing a Forbidden Emotion. Let's use crying as an example. When an emotional response involves crying, it often concerns the emotion of sadness. Pay attention the next time you cry in front of someone. Notice what you do physically. Likely you try to stop yourself from feeling this emotion by gulping, holding your breath, biting your lip, or any other way you can suppress your emotion.

A brilliant scene in the movie *Ordinary People* is a powerful illustration of this physical suppression. This scene takes a little over five minutes.

85

Donald Sutherland's character, Calvin, is in the dining room crying, feeling fully, and his wife, Beth, played by Mary Tyler Moore, comes downstairs to check on him. She asks him why he is crying, and she looks visibly uncomfortable with him emoting (Beth's suppression #1). She collects herself and asks him if she can get him something. He tells her she is determined, but not strong, and then he says he does not know if she is giving. You see this slight pressing together of her lips (Beth's suppression #2).

He then asks her if she loves him. Her response is that she feels the way she has always felt about him (Beth's suppression #3). Then he says they would have been all right if there had been no mess. He says that she cannot handle mess, that she needs everything neat and tidy. When he brings up their son Buck's death, emotion leaks out, but she immediately uses her mouth to suppress it again, by tightening her lips. (Beth's suppression #4).

When he tells her he does not know if he loves her anymore you see her inhale and then she purses her lips tight. She has practiced her suppression so much she stops herself from gasping (Beth's suppression #5). A hint of sadness surfaces that she immediately masks with anger as she presses her lips tightly once again. (Beth's suppression #6). Her eyes go blank as she turns around and heads upstairs, saying nothing (Beth's suppression #7).

When she enters the bedroom, she closes the door and lingers for a moment resting on the door yet still appearing stoic. She goes to the closet and once again lingers for a moment with both hands on the closet door before opening it. She takes her first suitcase, down off the shelf, appearing immovable emotionally. When she grabs the second suitcase from the closet it falls over making a loud noise that seems to startle her out of her suppression. She breaks down, as much as she can, but you see her fighting hard to not go too far down the emotional rabbit hole. She is falling apart inside and yet exerting a lot of effort to maintain control of her emotions. She is trying not to cry. It looks painful as she works to suppress her emotions (Beth's suppression #8).

How often do you allow yourself to feel fully? How often do you try to stop yourself from feeling, either through talking to yourself, taking physical action as Mary Tyler Moore's character did, or both? If you pay attention, you will find you do it more than you realize.

The Opposite of Feeling Fully

We live in a world where most of us are taught the opposite of feeling fully.

When you do not allow yourself to feel fully, emotional repression comes into play. If you have ever told yourself that you should *just think happy thoughts,* this creates more resistance as you attempt to repress whatever thoughts illicit the "not-so-happy thoughts."

Have you ever been caught in the whirl of an emotion? Perhaps you are angry with someone because they have said something unkind to you, and after the initial shock wears off and your Wounded Child emerges, your anger builds. You pace and mutter to yourself, things like:

"I don't believe them. How could they? What a bitch. What an asshole."

Then this other little, annoying voice, the Bully, gets loud, saying things like:

"Stop it. You need to be the bigger person here. Take the high road."

Don't believe this is the Bully? Pay attention to how uncomfortable it might feel for you to be angry. Pay attention to your self-talk. Notice the continuous mind chatter inside of you.

Do you try to make excuses for the other person?

Do you tell yourself you shouldn't feel this way?

Does something you heard about the downside of the emotion of anger pop into your head?

"Anger is a feeling that makes your mouth work faster than your mind." Author and humorist Evan Esar.

I'm sure you've heard the expression, "Never go to bed angry." But if you agree with your partner to never go to bed angry, what does that mean? Maybe you stay up late to resolve the issue, and then—because you are tired—you lash out. Then you feel bad and the Bully goes into overdrive with statements like:

"You should have kept your mouth shut."

"You just made it worse."

"What the hell were you thinking?"

"You just sunk to their level."

Blah blah blah blah blah!

Now how do you feel about yourself? I am betting even worse.

What if instead of trying to resolve the issue before going to bed, you gave your anger some space?

What if you soothed yourself by tapping on your anger, separate from the person you are angry with?

88

This is possible when you allow yourself your full-fledged anger while you use tapping to soothe your nervous system. By allowing yourself the space to do this and going to sleep without further discussion, you could wake up with more distance from your anger. You will then be less likely to lash out and more likely to say what you need to say in a clearer, more productive way.

In the above scenario you did not repress your anger. You allowed it in a much healthier way, which allowed you to move through it without all the added fall-out and regret of being in reaction mode.

The Dangers of Repression

On the flip side, maybe you say nothing to them. You just sit there and "take it." You are angry with a nice heaping helping of hurt, and you clamp down on your emotions. You feel like you can say nothing. When you leave the scene of the crime, you are whirling in an emotional stew that has no place to go. You ruminate on all the things you should have, or wish you would have, said to them. You head to the refrigerator and eat some ice cream, or grab a drink, or some other distraction that will soothe you. You do your best to suppress your anger and your hurt and go on with your day. A month later, you notice you have gained a few pounds and your anger turns more inward toward yourself.

Either scenario includes repression because both include some heavy-duty judgment. This judgment creates either emotional repression or acting out, and neither of these are healthy for you. If you feel hurt and angry because of something someone said to you and you do not have a healthy, effective way to deal with these feelings, you reject the emotional part of being human.

I call this trying to bypass your humanity. When this happens, you also bypass your creative energy, which allows you to receive guidance and direction on how to create a life you love. Another option is through spiritual bypass. This happens when you "try" to forgive, or "try" to take the high road or "try" to just let it go. Good luck! The emotion needs to go somewhere. Either option often ends up with you storing emotions in your body. They both create emotional repression.

How Emotional Repression Creates Forbidden Emotions

When growing up, you get bombarded with a lot of messages. You download thousands of messages, especially those from authority figures in your life. You might have the most inquisitive and curious mind, as all children do, but if you hear something often enough, you will likely believe it. Your resilience will wear down and the downloading begins. A lot of the messages you get are about emotions, specifically which emotions are "appropriate," and which are "forbidden."

This creates emotional repression. Trying to bypass your humanity, which means labeling yourself wrong for your human emotions, creates Forbidden Emotions. You try to repress them, and when you can no longer do so, your reactions are over-the-top. The same outcome occurs with spiritual by-passing.

Road rage is a perfect example of repressed emotions coming out in an over-the-top way.

Steve Albrecht, D.B.A., author of The Act of Violence, says in the article he wrote for Psychology Today, titled *"The Psychology of Road Rage: Anger and Violence Behind the Wheel."*

"What factors cause a usually mild-mannered person to see red? Some people who are ordinarily even-tempered admit that they have an easy tendency to lose control of their emotions when they get behind the wheel. Their fuses get lit when they put their keys into their ignitions.

For some road-ragers, it's a need for control, to counter to other drivers who they feel violate their proxemic space, or their need for possession of their lane or their part of the road. For others, it is unchecked anger and aggression. It's hormone-based, primitive, small-<u>brain</u> thinking, bringing a lack of <u>emotional intelligence</u> or the need to dominate someone else and their unsharable space. Add in unchecked egos, the need for superiority, <u>narcissistic</u> pride, and male genital one-upmanship: my vehicle is bigger than yours."

I will go out on a limb and say that the key ingredient here is the suppressed anger and aggression looking for an outlet. You find the outlet when someone cuts you off. You might be cool as a cucumber in other situations, but when driving you notice that your anger surfaces, so it surprises you and has you judging yourself.

Had they taught you a healthy, effective way to allow yourself to feel fully so you did not need to repress your emotions, you would be far less likely to carry around anger and aggression.

You could feel the feeling and allow it to move through you. You would be able to tell someone that you are angry, to own your anger and then deal with it, without the over-the-top expression of repressed emotions. I know from personal experience how liberating it is to tell someone I am angry and honor it and own it for myself and not let it get out of hand. It takes practice, and I believe it is always a work in progress you get better at.

What is the Harm of Forbidden Emotions?

Janice Berger, M.ED., a psychotherapist and lecturer on emotional health issues, says in her book Emotional Fitness, page 13 Published 2004:

> "When our natural emotional healing power is subverted, we do not complete feelings surrounding trauma and they stay buried within us. They become a reservoir of unfelt pain. Feelings are not buried dead; they are buried alive. They come up when we least expect them. They confuse and confound us. We control them in many different, destructive ways.

> Losing our real selves

> We learn as children, at a time when we are most vulnerable, to cry less than we need to, to be brave though we are fearful, to act as if anger does not exist. Gradually we lose touch with our feelings and by the time we are adults our sense of who we are is distorted. Our emotional health and our physical health are at risk."

She says that, "Each time we cannot feel an experience, tension develops."

So, where does this tension go? How does this buildup of tension get released? You can store it in your body and disease can develop. You can drive down the highway thinking you are fine when someone cuts you off or flips you off and BAM... you are off to the races and those buried emotions come out. You can go crazy and act out, even if there's no major consequence to anyone.

Who pays the price? You do, all over again, because it is likely you turned that anger on yourself by telling yourself you are crazy for reacting. Sometimes, other people pay a price as well because these scenes often end badly.

If you have ever heard a story about road rage where someone pulls a gun or runs someone off the road because they got cut off, you may marvel at how this could have happened. You might wonder what is wrong with someone who allowed themselves to get so out of control.

The more emotionally repressed someone is, the more depressed or aggressive they can get. Your emotions have to go somewhere; road rage is just one of many places. Your health can also suffer.

According to the US Department of Health and Human Services, "More than two-thirds (68.8 percent) of adults are considered overweight. Over one-third (35.7 percent) of adults are considered obese. Over 1 in 20 (6.3 percent) have extreme obesity. Almost 3 in 4 men (74 percent) are considered overweight or obese."

Having worked with many clients who suffer from obesity, we need to look beyond someone's diet to the underlying causes of obesity. The judgment in our society toward people who are obese is as much of an epidemic as being overweight is. In the work I do, I view weight as protection. Think about it this way: people gaining weight or carrying a lot of weight are virtually insulating themselves from others; they are creating a barrier between themselves and the outside world.

Debbie Shapiro talks about obesity in her book, *"The Body Mind Workbook"*:

"It puts a layer of fat between the inner self and the world, like a moat protecting us from fear of exposure, from being vulnerable and therefore hurt; yet it can equally stop us from freely expressing ourselves. Obesity often occurs after a great emotional shock or loss, as the emptiness experienced within us becomes too great to bear. This is the feeling of being empty of meaning or purpose, but our attempt to fill that emptiness causes more emptiness."

93

This is another cost of unfelt feelings and emotional repression; our bodies take on the burden of all the unfelt feelings we have buried. If you think about it this way, we have learned to reject our bodies, when they are supporting us and taking on our unexpressed emotions.

In my psychosomatic studies, or studies about the body/mind connection and how our unfelt feelings show up in our bodies, my teacher Carole Maureen Friesen always says:

"The issues are in our tissues."

When you learn to listen to your body, you learn the incredible intelligence of it. You can learn a lot about your internal world by paying attention to what is showing up in your health.

Remember my client, Mary, with an inoperable brain tumor that shrunk? Using her statement that doing work on her emotional blocks was the only thing she did differently. This dramatic healing can be evidence of the body/mind connection.

Louise Hay, creator of Hay House Publishing, wrote a New York Times best-selling book called, *"You Can Heal Your Life."* The following is from the About Louise L. Hay section of her book:

> In 1977 or 1978 she found she had cervical cancer, and she concluded that its cause was her unwillingness to let go of resentment over her childhood abuse and rape. She refused medical treatment, and began a regimen of forgiveness, therapy, reflexology, nutrition, and occasional enemas, and claims she rid herself of the cancer. She declared that there is no doctor left who can confirm this story but swore that it is true.

Whether or not you believe in the body/mind connection and how our emotions play a critical role in our state of health, you can find countless stories of people who have healed themselves of life-threatening illnesses through non-traditional means. Another story of body/mind healing comes from Anita Moorjani. She is a New York Times best-selling author of the book "*Dying to Be Me.*"

She says the following about being in a coma and in a near-death experience:

"I then started to understand how illnesses start on an energetic level before they become physical. If I chose to go into life, the cancer would be gone from my energy, and my physical body would catch up very quickly. I then understood that when people have medical treatments for illnesses, it rids the illness only from their body but not from their energy, so the illness returns. I realized if I went back, it would be with a healthy energy. Then the physical body would catch up to the energetic conditions very quickly and permanently. I seemed to become aware that this applies to anything, not only illnesses physical conditions, psychological conditions, etc. I became aware that everything going on in our lives was dependent on this energy around us, created by us. Nothing was real we created our surroundings, our conditions, etc. depending where this "energy" was. The clarity I felt around how we get what we do was phenomenal! It is all about where we are energetically. I somehow knew that I was going to see "proof" of this firsthand if I returned back to my body."

There are numerous stories about seemingly miraculous healing and the connection to our emotional bodies. When we bury emotions, they get buried in our bodies and can cause significant damage.

Types of Forbidden Emotions

A forbidden emotion is any emotion you do not allow yourself to feel—any emotion you judge yourself for feeling.

It could be an emotion like anger, for example, that your parents or caregivers forbade you to express and you downloaded that belief. Therefore, when you feel anger, you bury it. Perhaps you talk yourself out of it by saying things like, "I am not going to let him get to me," or you might automatically (subconsciously) use another emotion like guilt as a barrier against feeling the anger.

It could be an emotion like shame and your parents or caregivers might have encouraged it by saying things like, "Shame on you." However, because the emotion is so painful, you buried it, and it became a habit. Now when you feel shame, you still bury it. You may use food, alcohol, drugs, TV, being overly busy, or any other distraction. They may have wanted you to feel shame, but for you the pain of feeling it makes it forbidden for you. You might automatically use another emotion like anger as a barrier against feeling the shame.

It could be an emotion like hurt that your parents or caregivers neither discouraged nor encouraged, but because of the way it feels, you bury it. You might talk yourself out of it by saying things like, "She did not mean it when she said that," or you might automatically use another emotion like anger as a barrier against feeling the hurt.

Before I talk more about forbidden emotions, I want to talk more about self-judgment because we cannot change what we judge.

Self-judgment is a doozy. I find it can get missed in energy work. Self-judgment can be in your face, or it can be sneaky, or every variation between. Self-judgment is often accompanied by guilt, shame, despair, and more, and it is a defense against feeling those emotions. So, the first part of this work is to tap on the self-judgment to release some of it and get to those forbidden emotions.

I always say we learn to treat ourselves the way we were treated growing up. If you grew up with parents (it can be one or both) with high expectations for you, who expected you to be an achiever, to get straight A's, to live vicariously through you, that is a lot of pressure to live under. Imagine bringing home a B and facing their judgment? Maybe you do not have to imagine this.

Here is an "in your face" example:

I have a client who came close to fainting when she had to show her grades to her mother. She knew what was coming; the verbal beating she took for getting one B would put Buddha in a state of ill-repair. She learned to be hard on herself by her mother's example. This client has been an overachiever her entire life. She built a phenomenally successful business, but she never quite felt good enough. Her self-judgment was epic. She has had to practice unwinding her own brutality to herself.

Self-judgment can be very sneaky.

Here is a "sneaky" example:

You are looking at the dust bunnies floating around the living room. You know you "should" vacuum because you are having company tomorrow, but you just cannot bring yourself to do it because you are too comfortable on your couch binge-watching a Netflix series. The judgment begins. You may tell yourself that you are lazy for continuing to watch Netflix when you "should" be vacuuming. You do not get up and vacuum, but you feel this nagging guilt playing in your head like awful elevator music. You do not vacuum and yet you punish yourself by not enjoying the series you are watching. This is a lose-lose situation.

Self-judgment can also be comparing yourself to others. Whenever you compare, you lose. Anytime you tell yourself that you are wrong for feeling the way you do; you lock down on the behavior you want to release. It is hard to make changes around what you judge yourself over.

Here is a way to test this: think of something you do not like about yourself. As you call this to mind, pay attention to what you are saying to yourself. What is your self-talk?

It might sound like:

"I hate this about myself."

"I don't like this about myself."

"I'm so stupid."

You might even have a physical reaction when you think about it, cringing or shaking your head.

If you are judging yourself, notice how it feels in your emotional state and how it feels in your body to say the above statements. Does it feel heavy? When you are in self-judgment, it only creates more self-judgment because you lock down on whatever you are judging yourself for. You cannot change what you judge, so the cycle of self-judgment continues and gets worse as time goes on, but there is a way out of this cycle. It is about learning to love the part of you that judges you.

Now, with this same thing in mind, say to yourself:

"I want to love and accept the part of me that judges me."

Or:

"What if I can learn to love and accept the part of me that judges me?"

Notice the difference in your emotional state and how it feels in your body to say these statements. Does it feel lighter? Do you notice that your self-judgment has loosened just a little?

As you learn to become more in tune with your body, you will feel an enormous difference. If you are not feeling the difference, you're not doing anything wrong. This shift can take time. There is nothing wrong with you. The Bully might pipe up and try to tell you otherwise and just being aware of this, even without feeling a shift toward feeling a little lighter is a great first step. You may need to release more self-judgment with tapping to uncover that lightness. I will cover this in Chapter 5.

The next time you catch yourself using self-judgment, try using these softening, bridging statements.

"I'm open to accepting the part of me that judges me."

"What if the judge in me needs my acceptance as well?"

"It's good I'm aware of this because I can eventually soften and shift what I'm aware of."

When you practice this, you loosen your resistance, and when your resistance subsides, you are more likely to make positive changes.

Most of us have been wired to think by being hard on ourselves, we are more likely to change when the opposite is true.

When you practice softening your self-judgment, you will feel better, and when you feel better, you can be more of what you want to be and to act out of inspiration.

I will give you a personal example. I plan out my days. I have always chosen professions that have required planning on my part to do things. This means I push myself a lot. I can get caught up in what I call the "pushing" energy. I am pushing myself to complete things, and there's always self-judgment involved in this energy. I am a good person if I do it, and I am a bad person if I do not.

One day, I had my plan set. After finishing a client session, I had blocked out time to record my podcast, which was due the next day. It was time to do it, but I did not want to. I was pushing myself to do it. This felt heavy. My self-talk went something like, "Come on, Marti. It's due tomorrow. You've scheduled this time, so get it done." This all made rational sense, but I still did not want to do it. I had no idea what the topic would be, and I felt stuck.

Another part of me said, "Marti, go for a mountain bike ride."

"What?" I argued back. "It's 1:30 p.m. on a Thursday, and I need to get this done."

"Go for a mountain bike ride," the part said again.

I had a battle going. I was judging myself for even thinking about taking a mountain bike ride when I had work to do, but the truth was I felt better when I thought about taking the ride. So, I took the ride.

I felt like a kid. The sun was out, the air cool, a glorious day. I enjoyed the ride. I had released my self-judgment and chosen the path of joy and fun. Guess what happened while I was on the ride? The inspiration for my podcast came to me, and I was excited about it. When I got home, I felt inspired and creative, and I recorded, edited, and uploaded my podcast in less than 40 minutes.

I would not have had this inspiration had I stayed in self-judgment and pushed myself to do it. By releasing the judgment, I created the space for inspiration to come and then took inspired action. I felt joyful while out on my ride. I do my best now to follow the path of inspired action over the self-judging, pushing energy. It remains a work in progress.

The next time you catch yourself in self-judgment about what you should or should not do at the moment, go with what feels lighter, and see what happens. Do you feel better? Did you get a creative idea? Were you inspired in any way?

When you notice yourself feeling self-judgment about what you should have done or should have said about a past event, practice softening it and see what happens. This is tricky because the self-judgment is often a defense against feeling a forbidden emotion, but if you can remain curious and allow yourself to feel the feelings, you can release them. Stay with me because I will show you how.

But first, let's delve into some of the most common forbidden emotions.

Forbidden Emotion: Guilt

Guilt can have you curling up into a ball in the corner with a pacifier and a blanket, or you can bury guilt and do something like blame others or people-please to avoid feeling the guilt. Guilt is an indicator that something is off, and, in this way, it is helpful to us. The challenge is when guilt acts as a barrier to feeling and releasing other emotions.

When this happens, you become a guilty person, and you carry your unresolved guilt around with you.

When you allow yourself to feel guilt, depending on you and your past, it can lead to a variety of limiting beliefs and/or other emotions. When you do not allow yourself to feel through guilt, you do not get to feel what is under it, and you carry around unforgiven guilt.

When I say unforgiven, I mean you do not forgive yourself.

What to Do When You Have Wronged Someone Else

Here is an exercise:

Call to mind an event or situation where you believe that you wronged someone or where you behaved in a way you do not feel good about—something you feel guilty about. Do your best to tune in to a potential feeling related to this memory. When you feel like you are in touch with a feeling related to this event, say the following statement to yourself:

"I really forgive myself for this."

Rate how true this feels on the 0-10 scale. Zero means: I don't forgive myself. Ten means I forgive myself. Now say the statement again and ask yourself what emotion this brings up.

Rate how strong the emotion of guilt is on the 0 – 10 scale.

Now say these statements and rate how true they feel for you:

"I'm open to forgiving myself."
"I want to forgive myself."

If, through your rating, you realize that you are short on self-forgiveness, doing some forgiveness work can help move the dial for you emotionally so you can learn to practice more self-forgiveness. I will show you the best techniques I know for doing just this in the next chapter. Now let's try the reverse situation.

What to Do When Someone Has Wronged You

Call to mind an event or situation where you felt someone you love wronged you. This is where it gets interesting. Think about a parent, your partner, your sibling, or your child. Let's say you have a parent you believe wronged you when you were growing up, and you are now suffering consequences from this. Maybe you are angry with them, and yet you feel guilty for being angry with them. Here, guilt creates a barrier to allowing you to move through the anger you have buried. The guilt inhibits you from releasing the anger.

Say the following statement and instead of rating it, notice the self-talk that immediately follows you saying this.

"I'm right to be angry with them."

This might feel true that you have a right to be angry with them but notice if guilt surfaces. Most of us have a lot of programming about the dynamics with our parents.

Pay attention to how you feel when you are angry at a parent, a partner, or a child. Guilt is likely present on some level. You believe that your anger is inappropriate.

On Being Appropriate

When I work with clients who feel guilty because they are "not supposed to feel this way," we work on guilt first. This is often wrapped up in something called "being appropriate."

You can "be appropriate" to where you reject how you feel about a situation. When you do this, you do not have access to the emotion, and it stays buried in the body.

When working on the guilt these clients may feel about expressing their truth, I tell them to do their best to put being appropriate on the shelf temporarily and allow themselves to feel "inappropriate" emotions. I reassure them they can go back to being appropriate. The choice is theirs. Most people can do this. This allows the guilt to surface so we can attend to it. From there they can better allow their other emotions to surface.

You can learn to do this, which will allow for your own emotional healing.

When you allow yourself to feel your truth, you give your inner child a voice. During all the years you spent suppressing your emotions, you also suppressed the voice of the Wounded Child inside of you.

Think about yourself when you were little. How often were you encouraged to speak your truth? If you were not encouraged to do this, it is likely that you have Forbidden Emotions. You were told to be quiet, be appropriate, be a good girl or boy. This suppression of your truth, and your true feelings, resulted in suppressed emotions and suppressed potential. When you learn to give this part of you a voice, you open up a pathway for emotional liberation and freedom, and this opens up a world of possibility for you.

When you can attend to any guilt that comes up for you around speaking your truth in a healthy, safe, and productive way, you do a great service for not only yourself, but for those around you. You can also release shame along the way, which is our next Forbidden Emotion.

Forbidden Emotion: Shame

Shame is often a forbidden emotion, not because society forbids you to feel it, but because you have buried it. Shame is debilitating when you do not move through it. Parents, schools, and religious institutions all promote shame in their own ways. Think of:

"Shame on you."

"You should be ashamed of yourself."

Shame is a silent beast. It lurks in the background, gathering momentum and emotionally suffocating you, and this starts early in life. Think about what happened to you as a child. Children are amazing, vibrant beings, full-of-life, and you were likely just being your amazing, vibrant, full-of-life self when you got shamed into submission by being told to stop being so much you.

You could hear it in what was said to you. You could feel it running through your nervous system with a look from an authority figure. Shaming is learned, although some religions teach that you are born with original sin, which suggests infants come into this world shameful, it is up to you to decide what it true for you in this. I invite to consider how this makes you feel. Does it rob you of your joy, fun and enthusiasm to believe you are born sinful? If so, what might help you release some shame you may feel around this? Would it help to consider that you might not be inherently shameful?

Shame is like a glue in your energy system that binds other emotions to you. When you do not feel through it, it stays with you. It is like you live in a pool of it and it stops you from making progress. Shame must be felt through so you can move out of the shame pool.

Forbidden Emotion: Jealousy

If you have ever felt jealous of someone, it is likely that you have been taught that jealousy is unacceptable. You have probably been told that you should be happy for someone else's good fortune, but what do you do when you don't feel this way? Your inner Bully tells you this is "unacceptable," and the self-judgment and berating begins.

What do you do when you felt envious of someone? The next chapter will teach you how to deal with all of your Forbidden Emotions in the healthiest, safest way possible that I have found while working with my clients and myself.

Forbidden Emotion: Hatred/Anger/Rage

I put these three together because they are interrelated.

Hatred toward someone often surges because you feel powerless around this person. The person you feel hatred toward carries the power in the relationship, and you carry the victim energy. Let me add here I relate to this intimately. The more powerless I have felt in any relationship, the more powerful I found my hatred to be. This hatred turned to anger, which led to intense rage.

When I stopped arguing with my reality and stopped telling myself I should not feel emotions I was feeling, I allowed myself to feel my anger, hatred, and rage privately and fully while I tapped through it. I came out on the other side of it feeling liberated. I no longer felt the hatred; I replaced it with empathy for the person I directed my hatred at. That is a powerful transformation.

I had a client who felt intense hatred toward a family member she felt disempowered around. When we tapped together on her hatred and she went into it and ranted it out, I could hear it turning to anger and then to intense rage as we tapped, and she continued to allow herself to feel her emotions. I told her to keep tapping and to let it spill out of her as much as she could. She kept tapping as the feelings intensified and she let them come up and out. She said it astonished her at how much rage her hatred of this family member caused her to feel. It was the first time she'd let herself feel so fully, and after session, she felt a huge releasing of energy.

Later that week, I got an email from her saying she could not believe the change in her behavior. She had spoken to the family member the day after our session and instead of getting triggered, she laughed. She felt it was a miracle. She had never had this reaction before. She felt so much freer. This is the power of feeling fully.

Forbidden Emotion: Hurt

Hurt is another emotion some of us do not allow ourselves to feel because, well, it hurts, and it makes us feel small and weak. Some of us feel anger instead of hurting. Hurt is often the layer under anger, especially if we feel betrayed.

I have found that some people automatically go to hurt and have difficulty feeling anger, while other people automatically feel anger and have difficulty feeling hurt.

If you get triggered easily and automatically feel hurt, it is often because you have left over hurt from the past.

If you get triggered easily and automatically feel anger, there's often hurt under the anger—also from the past—and you have made hurt a forbidden emotion.

Tapping will help you wade through hurt and anger from the past.

Forbidden Emotion: Joy

You might wonder how a desirable feeling like joy can be a Forbidden Emotion. Here is how: When you have things happening in your life you are excited about, you may feel you have to downplay how joyful or happy you feel about what is happening for you, especially around people not as fortunate. This is when joy or happiness becomes forbidden to you; you put a lid on your joy, so others do not feel bad.

The Upside of Forbidden Emotions

I just touched on a few emotions here, but you can pick any emotion and find a way for it be forbidden. I see this because of my work in the personal development field, and because of what I see happening in my life and the lives of people I have had the privilege of working with. Your life can change for the better when you embrace your amazing full palette of emotions by allowing them to move through your body to their completion. Tapping can help you do this.

You have these emotions for a reason. If you go back to Abraham Hicks Emotional Guidance Scale, the entire premise is that your emotions are your guidance. They tell you where you are at and how connected you are to yourself through your emotional landscape.

When you learn to feel fully and embrace the amazing guidance your emotions give you, you will show up differently for the most important person in your life: you. A by-product of this is that you become much more effective in your relationships with others. Once you learn the art of self-acceptance, you can affect true, lasting change, and the best way you can practice self-acceptance is with your emotions.

As you allow yourself to feel your forbidden emotions more fully, you release them from your energy system.

They are no longer buried alive in you, as Janice Berger says in Emotional Fitness. They no longer come out at inopportune times, and you learn to become more present with yourself.

Years ago, I heard actress Debrah Farentino talk about what she loved about acting in an interview. She said something that stood out for me. She said, "In acting, you get to say just the right thing, at just the right moment, which you seldom get to do in real life."

I loved that. How often do you get to do this in real life? This is a huge upside to feeling fully. You will learn to be more present with yourself and, because of this, you will give yourself more time to feel and then respond from a conscious place instead of reacting unconsciously.

As you learn there are not any forbidden emotions, you will embrace all of your emotions more fully and become more emotionally intelligent. You might still react to something, but your ability to catch yourself in the act allows you to have more choice around how far you will go into an emotion. As you soothe yourself with tapping, this allows to you respond more than react. There will also be times when you can intentionally use an emotion.

For example, one time, after I got our dog, Luci, we were out hiking, and I heard her whimper behind me. I turned around to see four coyotes following her. She had sense enough to know that they intended harm to her, so she found me and came up right next to me. I thought to myself, "Well, this would be an excellent time to call upon my rage and use it to get rid of these coyotes." So, I did just that. I called upon my inner rage and did the best pissed-off grizzly bear imitation I could muster and let me say, those four coyotes ran off faster than a speeding bullet. This was an intentional use of rage.

Other times, rage will just spring up without us intentionally trying to use it. Rage will spring up because of, say, a perceived injustice. The rage is the guidance telling you there is an injustice, and when you accept rage as a natural emotion to experience, there's no second guessing if you should feel rage or not.

This is the rule of thumb for dealing with your variation of Forbidden Emotions. When you notice yourself feeling bad about whatever you are feeling, it is a strong indicator you are judging yourself for whatever you are feeling. Let yourself feel what you feel. Working toward self-acceptance is key. This takes practice. Learning of your self-judgment takes practice.

Awareness is the first step and acceptance is the second. Acceptance is tough at first. We have been programmed to judge ourselves, and we notice all the ways we judge ourselves. A self-judgment can be as simple as, "I should forgive them," to a more severe version, "I'm such a horrible person because I hate them." Sometimes we hate. Sometimes it is too soon to forgive.

Most of us do not want to stay in hatred or non-forgiveness, but when we judge it, we cannot change it. As we learn of these feelings and learn to own and accept them, we can then change the ways they affect us, by realizing they're just emotions.

It's important to remind yourself often that you will be a lifelong work in progress; there is no getting to "I am perfect now." I do not know about you, but when I realized that, I felt such great relief. I did not have to fix myself today for a better tomorrow.

Here is another personal example that shows the power in managing your emotions.

I had an argument with a friend. We were getting scrappier by the minute, but when I went down the rabbit hole of emotion, I caught myself. I stopped and went into the bathroom to collect myself because I knew that I did not want to keep heading in this direction. The only thing I could do was manage myself, and I knew I did not want to keep hurting myself. I could control nothing going on with the other person, and I was not attached to having to do that. I left the bathroom, went up to my friend, and said, "I am sorry for my part in this. I know I was getting crazy with this, but I don't want to now, and I'm sorry for what I said."

My friend, who was having none of it, gave me the finger and said, "Fuck you," and I was astonished not by what my friend did, but because I got it. I had been there myself. I was amazed at how calm I felt. I just thought to myself, "This person is not ready." So, I grabbed my purse and left. I waited about an hour before I texted my friend and said, "You may not be anywhere near unfuck you, but when you are, I'm willing to talk." My friend called me immediately and said, "I am sorry. That was uncalled for. I was still just too angry."

These are magical moments for me, when I am in a place of wanting to free myself from my madness. I was not judging myself for my behavior. I accepted and forgave myself, and the upside of this embracing of my emotions was that I did not judge my dysfunctional actions in the same way. I was aware I did not want to continue down that path, and I dealt with it in the healthiest way I could. When handled this way, the other people you are dealing with can often free themselves, too.

By releasing emotional blockages in a safe and healthy way, and by allowing yourself to feel fully, you learn to allow emotions to move through you freely, as they should do.

You will find the more you embrace and release these buried Forbidden Emotions, the freer you feel emotionally. You can better manage your emotional state and soothe yourself by soothing your nervous system. You can better handle the ups and downs of life without feeling so overwhelmed.

Your emotions no longer run your show. Instead, they guide you. When your emotions no longer run your show, you make better decisions because you have learned to pull yourself out of fight-or-flight mode. You release chronic emotional stress, and you will find more often than not that you can do what actress Debrah Farentino spoke about, by having just the right response at just the right moment.

I want to point out here sometimes, you may never have the right response, and that is okay, too. I used to beat myself up for not having the right response until I realized that sometimes, there is no right response. Sometimes, no matter what you say, your words might be taken the wrong way, or set someone off. Even if ninety-nine out of 100 people think it is the right response, you might be talking to that 100th person. Be compassionate with yourself and try to accept that it is okay to not always have the right response.

As you release the limiting beliefs that got installed in your operating system when you were a young child, there's an amazing benefit to allowing all your emotions to be just as they are, without judgment. As you demonstrate emotional intelligence because you are clearing out your emotional clutter, you remember who you are. You notice intuitive thoughts more often, and you understand this intuitive thought is your guide.

I heard a great story years ago when I lived in Chicago. I went to a talk at my church by Jerry Jampolsky and Diane Cirincione (https://www.miraclecenter.org/wp/about/people/gerald-and-diane/).

They talked a lot about *A Course in Miracles, by Helen Schucman* which contains a curriculum to bring about what it calls a "spiritual transformation."

They shared a story of a couple with a toddler and a new baby. The toddler requested that they allow him to be alone with the baby in the baby's room. The parents were concerned because they thought maybe their son was jealous of the baby, and they could not understand why he was so insistent on having time alone with the baby. They came up with allowing him to be alone with the baby with the baby monitor on so they could hear if anything were amiss.

Once the boy was in the room alone with his baby sibling, he said, "Baby, teach me about God. I'm beginning to forget."

When I heard this, it gave me chills. I believe that when we are born, we are fresh from our source, whatever that source may be for you. We come with everything already installed in us. There's nothing missing. We understand our Divine Nature, and it is not in words; it is in understanding. As we become more indoctrinated into our human incarnation, however, we forget who we are. We forget that everything we need is already within us. We forget that we have a direct line to the Creator, always; it never leaves us. It is not about pulling more into us; it is about removing the emotional stew covering over our Divine Nature.

As you find yourself freer of the emotions that get stuck in your energy system, you will remember. You will notice more intuitive sensitivity. You will remember you are your own best expert.

When my daughter was just a couple of months old, we would put her in a baby swing. I would wind it up and watch her be rocked back and forth by the motorized swing. She would immediately look upward and coo and giggle and talk baby talk. I had no idea what she was saying, but I used to say to her dad, "She's talking to the angels again." I believe she was talking to something divine, communing with higher energies. She was always happy and smiling and in such a state of joy. I am convinced she was in the presence of Divine Energy. It brought me joy to watch her. She was fresh from Spirit, so unencumbered by the trappings of humanity.

This is also true of my oldest sister, who had brain surgery when she was 9 years old. Because of the tumor and resulting surgery, she had damage to her brain and was considered mentally handicapped. She always saw the best in everyone. If you met her, she would have given you a genuine compliment right away. She was a joy-spreader. She experienced a wide range of emotions, but she was not bogged down by the same emotional trappings that most of humanity is. Her mind was not in the way of her experiencing joy and kindness. A friend puts it this way: "She's had a pure heart." I would agree. She was more in touch with her truth as a Divine Being. She preached the religion of love, without trying too. It's who she was. It's in all of us. She was freer of all of life's human trappings, so she was in touch with her Divine Nature.

As you learn to free yourselves from the ties that bind you emotionally, you return to a state like the one I witnessed with my daughter when she was a baby, and the one my sister enjoyed her entire life.

You remember your true essence—your Divine Nature. You no longer have to be positive or try so hard anymore. You rekindle the excitement and enthusiasm you had as a little child before the limiting downloads.

Now... how do you get there? That is what the rest of this book is about.

Chapter Summary

Forbidden Emotions are any emotion you tell yourself are not okay to feel.

It's the emotions you attempt to shut down on.

They're off limits. You know you're experiencing forbidden emotions when you tell yourself you shouldn't be feeling whatever you're feeling. This creates repression of emotion which creates tension in the body, which has the potential to weaken your immune system due to chronic elevated cortisol levels in your body.

As you learn to open yourself up to these emotions and use a safe and healthy tool like tapping to release them, you can find that every area of your life improves. You also learn how to be true to yourself and say what you need to say in circumstances, where in the past you might have "put up and shut up."

This is a great example of self-care. Learning to value yourself and all of your emotions first. You put *you* first and by doing this, you are giving other people permission to do the same without judgment.

The Basics of Tapping

I will use the term "Tapping" throughout the rest of this book in place of Emotional Freedom Techniques, or EFT.

This chapter will review the basics of Tapping. In the following sections, I will discuss tapping from my perspective. A perspective formed from the thousands of sessions I have done with clients and from what I have found to be robust and effective ways to use tapping.

If you are unfamiliar with Tapping, be prepared for a surprising, slightly strange, and yet highly effective energy medicine technique. One with the power and potential to change your life for the better. Once you experience results from this technique, you will feel more confident in it, no matter how strange it may seem at first.

What Is Tapping?

Tapping is a form of energy psychology. It is a cross between acupuncture and modern-day psychology. You use your fingertips instead of needles to tap on and stimulate Chinese acupuncture points, also known as meridian points.

Kootenay Columbia College of Integrative Health Science in Nelson, British Columbia, Canada who offers a 5-year Doctor of Traditional Chinese Medicine Program that requires over 4005 hours of course work and many other programs and training. Their definition of meridians is:

"Simply put, a meridian is an 'energy highway' in the human body. Qi (chee) energy flows through this meridian or energy highway, accessing all parts of the body. Meridians can be mapped throughout the body; they flow within the body and not on the surface,

117

meridians exist in corresponding pairs and each meridian has many acupuncture points along its path.

The term 'meridian' describes the overall energy distribution system of Chinese Medicine and helps us to understand how basic substances of the body (Qi, blood, and body fluids) permeate the whole body. The individual meridians themselves are often described as 'channels' or even 'vessels' which reflects the notion of carrying, holding, or transporting qi, blood and body fluids around the body."

Tapping works within this system. There are scientific studies behind this technique to prove its efficacy.

Dr. David Feinstein, a clinical psychologist, is an internationally recognized leader in the rapidly emerging field of energy psychology. His research papers have provided a foundation for understanding how it is possible to quickly and non-invasively alter brain chemistry for therapeutic gain. His award-winning, popular books have opened the approach to many.

The following comes directly from Dr. Feinstein's website:

Energy Psychology has been called "acupressure for the emotions." By tapping energy points on the surface of the skin while focusing the mind on specific psychological problems or goals, the brain's neural pathways can be shifted to quickly help you:

Overcome Fear, Guilt, Shame, Jealousy, Anger, or Anxiety

Change Unwanted Habits and Behaviors Enhance the Ability to Love, Succeed, and Enjoy Life

He also adds this on the EFT Universe Website:

"A literature search identified 51 peer-reviewed papers that report or investigate clinical outcomes following the tapping of acupuncture points to address psychological issues. The 18 randomized controlled trials in this sample were critically evaluated for design quality, leading to the conclusion that they consistently demonstrated strong effect sizes and other positive statistical results that far exceed chance after relatively few treatment sessions. Criteria for evidence-based treatments proposed by Division 12 of the American Psychological Association were also applied and found to be met for a number of conditions, including PTSD." [5]

If you want to learn more about his journey from skepticism, I recommend you read *The Promise of Energy Psychology: Revolutionary Tools for Dramatic Personal Change*. Dr. Feinstein co-wrote this book with Donna Eden and EFT Founder Gary Craig.

On my own journey with EFT, I dove in, used it, and noticed a difference within a few months.

Understanding the Basics of Tapping

Let's start by going over the tapping points.

Here is a tapping chart so you can see the tapping points:

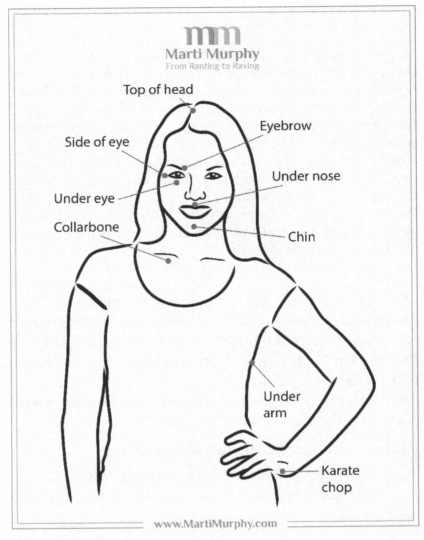

I will go through each point and explain each exercise.

Karate Chop Point:

This is where we begin. It is literally the side of the hand you would use to karate chop a board. When tapping, you will tap your karate chop point continuously while saying the set-up phrases, which I will discuss as well (see included diagram).

120

Tapping Point Sequence (Following Karate Chop):
Eyebrow
Side of the eye
Under the eye
Under the nose
Chin point
Collarbone
Under the arm
Top of the head
(See included diagram)

Now that you are familiar with the tapping points, I will explain how to use them.

Step One: Choose a Target

We start with a target. This can be an emotion, a memory of an event, a symptom, or a limiting belief. For simplicity,

Examples of each target:

An Emotion – What emotion do you feel about a memory of an event, a symptom, or a limiting belief? Are you angry, enraged, sad, frustrated, irritated, impatient, afraid, doubtful, disappointed, jealous, grieving, depressed, in despair, overwhelmed, bored, discouraged, insecure, guilty, or worried? Choose the emotion/feeling that most closely matches where you are at. Let's say you are aware you are feeling sad. You would start with the statement, "I feel sad."

A Memory of an Event – When you recall an event that happened to you, it could be about the friend who teased you. It could be when you asked your boss for a raise. It could be the memory of when you and your boyfriend or girlfriend broke up, etc. These are examples of a memory of an event. Sometimes you can be in touch with a feeling around it and sometimes not. Either way, it does not matter, as you will tap on the event, or the story and emotions can surface and even change from one emotion to another.

A Symptom – Symptoms are things like face twitches, rashes, digestion issues, sore throat, respiratory infections, coughing, stomach aches or crapping, leg cramps, eye-watering, eye infection, etc.

A Limiting Belief – You notice your income never increases, or you can never seem to find a lasting partnership, or your bosses are always challenging for you to deal with. Look at what is showing up in your life. If it is something you continue to struggle with, it is a good indicator you have a limiting belief in place. It has you repeating the same or similar circumstances in your life that aren't working for you.

Step Two: Rate Your Target

Once we have a target in mind, we move on to the subjective units of distress (SUDs) scale. The SUDs scale is a 0 – 10 scale. You rate how strong the emotion or emotional charge connected to an event feels, how intense a symptom feels, or how true a limiting belief feels.

For example:

You have a memory of a fight you had with your mother. When you call this event to mind, you need to tune in to the emotion behind the fight you had. As you bring the event to mind, what emotion comes to the forefront? If you do not know, try guessing. I always ask clients, "If you had to guess, what emotion do you think you feel?" It is incredible how they can always come up with an emotion when guessing. My belief is that since they are not as attached to the emotion at that moment, it comes to mind more freely.

Say, for example, the emotion is anger. I find it's helpful to use a statement such as: "I'm angry with my mother about our fight."

Now you want to use the SUDs scale to rate how strong the anger feels when you call to mind the fight with your mother.

0 = Not angry at all

10 = Extremely angry

Let's say you choose an eight. This indicates the intensity of your anger when you call to mind this event with your mother.

Do your best to trust what is coming to you when tapping. Aim to intuit what rating feels right to you and go with it. At first, it may seem foreign or awkward, but the more you do it, the more efficiently your intuition will supply the rating.

If you try to intellectualize what number you "should" feel, pause and instead answer this question: "If you had to guess how angry you are on a scale of 1–10, what would it be?" Like the similar question about emotion above, this allows space so a rating can come more freely.

If the SUD's scale doesn't resonate with you, just notice how heavy it feels in your body.

Step Three: Recite Your Set-Up Statements

Set-up statements are statements you use for setting your brain up to tap. You are letting your conscious and subconscious mind know that you have a challenge. Still, you accept, or at least acknowledge, yourself anyway. To get started, you tap on the karate chop point while repeating the set-up statement 3 times.

The set-up statements start with *"Even though..."* and are recited while tapping on the karate chop point. A set-up statement might sound like this:

While tapping on the karate chop point: *"Even though I'm really angry with my mother about our fight, I accept myself anyway."*

I tell clients to tune in to what feels truest for them. For some people, saying they accept themselves does not feel right. This is where Forbidden Emotions show up. Deep down, you think, "I'm not supposed to be angry, and I'm definitely not supposed to be angry with my mother." We'll talk about this more later in this chapter, but for now, if you do not feel accepting of yourself and your feelings, here are examples of options that can feel truer:

Karate chop tapping: "Even though I'm angry with my mother about our fight, I acknowledge myself and my feelings anyway."

Karate chop: "Even though I'm angry with my mother about our fight, I want to accept myself anyway."

Karate chop: "Even though I'm angry with my mother about our fight, I want to want to accept myself even if I don't right now."

These variations may help the set-up statements feel truer. I encourage you to change the wording as you need to and instead say something like:

"I acknowledge myself and my feelings..."

"I want to accept myself..."

"I want to want to accept myself, even if I don't right now..."

Quick Review

Set-up statements begin with saying, *"Even though..."* They are used while tapping on the karate chop point, and they are repeated three times.

After tapping on the set-up statement three times, you move to the reminder phrases.

Step Four: Add Reminder Phrases

Reminder phrases should remind you about what you are tapping to clear. You tap through the tapping points, starting at the eyebrow, as you say these statements.

Example:

Eyebrow: I am really angry with my mother.

Side of the eye: I do not like feeling this way, but I do.

Under the eye: I am furious about our fight.

Under the nose: I do not like being angry about this.

Chin point: I tell myself I should not feel angry, but I do.

Collarbone: I am just so angry right now.

Under the arm: I do not want to stay angry, but right now, I am.

Top of the head: I feel a lot of anger about this.

You would continue to repeat this tapping sequence starting at the eyebrow and continuing with what feels right for you. These are often called negative statements, but a nicer way to look at them is that you are tapping on what feels right for you, and that can often feel negative to you. You would continue to tap on what feels right for you for around 6–8 rounds. Longer if needed.

Then you would go back to the SUDs scale and rate your feeling of anger again. It is always helpful to ask a question, like:

"Am I angry with my mother about our fight?"

0 = Not angry at all

10 = Extremely Angry

You would rate it again and see if the number has dropped from your original score to a lower number.

Do not Fear Fluctuating Ratings

Ratings can go up and down with tapping. Often the number goes down; however, sometimes the feelings intensify. That is why we do 6–8 tapping rounds. I tell my clients before we tap that their feelings may intensify with tapping. That is a good thing because it means we have targeted the emotion. Trust the tapping to do what it is supposed to do; soothe your nervous system, ease the fight-or-flight response, and keep tapping through the sequences provided. You will get relief; it is just that sometimes it requires you to tap longer on your target.

Once your nervous system soothes, your numbers will go down.

Next, you want to bring in positive bridging statements.

Step Five: Transition to Positive Bridging Statements

Here is an example of positive bridging statements:

Eyebrow: What if it is okay to feel angry?

126

Side of the eye: It is just a feeling anyway.

Under the eye: What if I don't stay angry about this?

Under the nose: Time does make a difference.

Chin point: What if I can get through this and move on?

Collarbone: What if feeling angry is okay?

Under the arm: What if the first step is to accept myself and my feelings right where I am now?

Top of the head: What if through acceptance, I can move through this anger faster?

These bridging rounds help to move you toward feeling better because they help your brain to believe them more readily than definitive statements. They help to bridge your thoughts to a better feeling place.

How Tapping Helps Uncover Forbidden Emotions

Let's go back to the set-up statements. This is where you can uncover Forbidden Emotions immediately. When you have resistance to saying you accept yourself, your feelings, or what you are experiencing, this is a psychological newsflash that you are dealing with Forbidden Emotions.

Using the example of being angry at your mother, think about all the programming around parents.

Honor Thy Father and Mother

Children Should Be Seen and Not Heard

Father Knows Best

Respect Your Elders

What do you do when your mother or father doesn't behave honorably, or your father doesn't know best?

What if your parent gives you the silent treatment for making a mistake?

What if your elder's own Wounded Child is running their show on a particular day and you suffer because of that?

What if your parents won't listen to your side of the story?

What if your mother demanded more from you than you felt capable of?

Does this make them right? Does this mean that no matter what their behavior, you are supposed to honor and respect them?

> *"Parents are the ultimate role models for children. Every word, movement, and action have an effect. No other person or outside force has a greater influence on a child than the parent."*
>
> ~ *Bob Keeshan (Captain Kangaroo)*

Think of anyone you know who is in a position of authority. Because they hold a position of authority, does this automatically make them right? Think about this because this is the programming that many of us get. Many people on this planet in positions of authority misbehave. Are you supposed to respect and honor them anyway?

This is where Forbidden Emotions first get installed.

You are told to respect your elders, but were you taught to decide for yourself what feels right and true for you?

When you are told to respect someone who does not behave respectfully, witnessing this as a child can be the ultimate mind-mess.

You know something's off. You know something doesn't feel right, but you are "just a child," so what do you know? You learn over time to doubt yourself and tell yourself you are wrong for being angry if you are told you should not be.

It is crazy making to tell a child they should not feel what they are feeling. That goes for us adults, too.

So how can Tapping help you uncover and release Forbidden Emotions?

Remember that in tapping, we begin with choosing a target, which means to select an emotion, an event, a symptom, or a limiting belief. Let's go back to the example of being angry with your mother. Say you put a lid on your anger or make excuses for any behavior she did that felt inappropriate to you. You do this because she is your mother, and you have a belief that it is not okay to be angry with her. This reluctance to feel what you are feeling tells you that you are dealing with a Forbidden Emotion.

Here is why: you are angry, but you tell yourself you "should not" be, so you cut off the anger without feeling it and thus without processing through it. This emotion then gets frozen in your energy system, or as Janice Berger stated in Emotional Fitness, "It gets buried alive."

When this happens, you are stuck with the belief you "should not" get angry with her, or that you "should" just let it go. You "should" just get over it because she is your mother. This creates a barrier to allowing the emotion to do what it is intended to do: move through you.

Any time you tell yourself you "should not" feel angry, or sad, or anything you are feeling, no matter what the emotion, you are dealing with Forbidden Emotions.

The Challenge of Unprocessed Feelings

What happens with unprocessed feelings? They surface at some of the most inappropriate times. If you have had an experience, with yourself or someone else, where the surfacing emotion seems "over-the-top," it is because you, or they, are dealing with a Forbidden Emotion.

Any unprocessed emotions are forbidden because somewhere along the way you were told or given a look or some other indication to stop feeling whatever you were feeling.

With tapping, you are activating neural pathways in the brain attached to the target you chose, so the unprocessed emotions surface. As you tap, you allow yourself to process these emotions so they can be released.

In Chapter 3, I mentioned a phrase one of my mentors, EFT Master Carol Look, often uses when working with someone:

"My parents did the best they could, but it sucked for me."

The first time I heard her say this, I loved it. I felt like it summed up how I felt. It was such a relief because, when my anger came out of my childhood, I always tried to quell it with this refrain*: "No matter what happened, my parents did the best they could."*

While this is true, they did do their best, I also needed to honor my experience. To allow myself to express and release how angry I felt about what happened. I could not do this while deferring my emotions and focusing on this refrain instead.

Until I acknowledged how heartbroken and sad I was, without telling myself I should not feel that way, my anger and sadness stayed buried within me.

I will come back to this example in the next chapter on Rant Tapping. I will show you how to use Rant Tapping effectively and safely to release entrenched Forbidden Emotions.

For now, let's review the basics of tapping.

Review: 5 Steps to Tapping on a Target

Here are the steps to take for each tapping session:

1) Choose a target: an event, an emotion, a symptom, a limiting belief.
2) Rate your target on the SUDs scale of 0–10.

3) Start with the set-up statements. Repeat your "Even though..." statement 3 times while
tapping on the karate chop point.

4) Move to the tapping points with reminder phrases.

> Eyebrow
> Side of the eye
> Under the eye
> Under the nose
> Chin point
> Collarbone
> Under the arm
> Top of the head

5) Transition to positive bridging statements to help move you toward feeling better.

Example:

I had just finished my EFT Levels 1 and 2 Certification Training in Chicago and had flown back to Albuquerque. My husband picked me up at the airport. An interesting dynamic occurred for us when we would come back together after being apart, many sometimes we would get into an argument.

When he picked me up this time, I had a lot of anxiety, but I had no idea why. I am sure my awareness was heightened because I had just completed six intense days of training. I said nothing to him. Before learning about tapping, I would have been unconscious of what I was feeling. Let me add that tapping has helped me to identify my feelings more readily. I am no longer as confused or frozen around my emotions.

He had a few things to do but said he would drop me off at our house to let me get settled, and then he would come back and pick me up to go to lunch. I was relieved for the time alone to uncover what was behind my anxiety.

After he dropped me off, I tapped on my feeling of anxiety. Before I knew it, a memory from childhood surfaced that before this, I had no conscious recollection of.

It was a memory of my parents fighting, and one had threatened to leave the other. My sisters lined up to get on the phone with my mom, who was staying at a hotel, and my father was on the phone with her. She apparently wanted to talk to each of us.

As I watched my sisters waiting to talk to her, I noticed something in this memory. It was how anxious I felt watching each sister take their turn getting on the phone with my mother. My mother was upset, as was my father.

I kept tapping through this memory as the tears flowed. I trusted the tapping to do what it is meant to do: help me process those unprocessed emotions until the anxious feelings dissipated. I felt tired but relieved at the end of this tapping.

When my husband came back to pick me up, I shared with him what had happened, and we had a pleasant lunch.

When I tell people this example, they often ask, *"How did the anxiety you felt when your husband picked you up at the airport relate to that memory?"*

I'm not entirely sure, but in my EFT training, I was told about a thing in tapping called "linking." Essentially this means that memories with a similar emotional charge get linked in neuron clusters in the neural pathways in our brains. This is why when you tap, you can have a memory surface that, from a rational perspective, makes no sense as to why it surfaced, given the target you were tapping on.

I tell clients that our brains are amazing. They bring up what needs to be brought up to process emotions so we can release them from our energy system. When clients know this, they are better able to allow the process to unfold organically.

Below are basic tapping scripts to get you started.

132

Please take responsibility for yourself when tapping. Having intense emotions surface is a good thing because it means you have targeted an unprocessed emotion and are now releasing it.

While tapping through these, tune in to how you are feeling when tapping. Notice if you tell yourself you should not feel something, or you should not say something out loud. Noticing your self-talk is an excellent barometer as to whether or not you are dealing with Forbidden Emotions.

These general tapping scripts can get you in touch with when you are telling yourself you "should not" have particular emotions.

Disclaimer:
There are more tapping sequences in this chapter, so know that strong emotions can surface, and this indicates that we have targeted an emotion. Please take responsibility for yourself and keep tapping until you feel soothed. Always consult your therapist or medical doctor before going through these exercises.

You find this because tapping can effectively help you to release and neutralize these potently forbidden thoughts, experiences, and emotions within you anyway. A possible and even likely outcome is you experience true emotional freedom, perhaps even genuine compassion, forgiveness, and peace without having to try. Compassion and forgiveness are often natural by-products of feeling fully; expressing, and thus releasing, what has been seen as forbidden.

How to Tap on Anger

Work your way through this entire segment, tapping on the point listed on the left as you say the corresponding statement out loud.

Karate chop point: Even though I should not feel angry, it is really not okay, I acknowledge I feel this way.

Karate chop: Even though I should not feel angry, I accept that I have this belief.

Karate chop: Even though I have this belief that anger is not okay, I deeply and profoundly accept myself anyway.

Eyebrow: I should not feel angry.

Side of the eye: It is a destructive emotion.

Under the eye: I refuse to feel angry.

Under the nose: It is just not a good emotion.

Chin point: It is not okay to feel angry.

Collarbone: I have tons of evidence to prove this is true.

Under the arm: I should not feel angry.

Top of the head: But sometimes I just do.

Eyebrow: I need to stop feeling it.

Side of the eye: I need to not express it.

Under the eye: I should not let it out.

Under the nose: I should just let it go.

Chin point: It is not okay to feel angry.

Collarbone: I need to let this go.

Under the arm: It is bad to feel angry.

134

Top of the head: Is it really?

Eyebrow: Where did I learn that anger is bad?

Side of the eye: That I should not feel it.

Under the eye: What if anger is just an emotion?

Under the nose: What if it is essential to express anger healthfully and productively?

Chin point: What if by allowing myself to express it, I am better able to release it?

Collarbone: And truly let it go.

Under the arm: What if tapping through this anger is a healthy way to express and release it?

Top of the head: What if I am better off expressing it this way?

Eyebrow: I do not have to direct my anger to someone's face.

Side of the eye: I can do it privately right now and at least take the edge off of it.

Under the eye: What if allowing myself to feel my anger this way really helps?

Under the nose: What if by allowing myself to feel my anger while tapping, I can get to a better place?

Chin point: What if I can learn over time how to express my anger without the drama?

Collarbone: What if it is just an emotion?

Under the arm: What if by expressing my anger this way...

Top of the head: Over time, I am better able to handle my emotions?

Eyebrow: What if I am doing myself a favor?

Side of the eye: What if the more I tap through my anger, the less angry I feel?

Under the eye: What if I am better able to communicate my anger healthfully?

Under the nose: What if this is better for me and better for everyone?

Chin point: What if by feeling fully, I become the best version of myself?

Collarbone: What if I do not have to be afraid of my anger anymore...

Under the arm: Because I now have a healthy and productive way to feel and release...

Top of the head: As I am intended to.

Take a breath.

Rate how strong the feeling is now, from 0 (not strong at all) to 10 (extremely strong).

If the feeling is stronger, it means you have targeted the emotions. Go back and do the tapping sequence as often as you need to until you feel soothed, and these negative statements feel less true for you. This is a great indicator you are moving in the right direction.

How to Tap on Sadness

Work your way through this entire segment, tapping on the point listed on the left as you say the corresponding statement out loud.

Karate chop: Even though I feel this sadness and it is uncomfortable for me, I love and accept myself anyway.

Karate chop: Even though I feel sad and I am not sure why, but I know I feel it, I accept myself and my feelings now.

Karate chop: Even though this sadness feels like it has been in me a long time, I acknowledge myself right now.

Eyebrow: I feel this sadness.

Side of the eye: It is not comfortable, but I feel it.

Under the eye: I feel it in my body.

Under the nose: I have felt this before, and it is not something I like to feel.

Chin point: I just feel sad right now.

Collarbone: I feel sad.

Under the arm: I feel like a little child, too.

Top of the head: What if it is okay to feel this?

Eyebrow: This sadness in me...

Side of the eye: What if it is not comfortable, but it is really okay?

Under the eye: What if just acknowledging the sadness is a good first step?

Under the nose: Feeling fully is not something I was taught to do well.

Chin point: What if this is just like learning a new language?

Collarbone: I am learning the language of feelings.

Under the arm: What if there's a big benefit to feeling and releasing?

Top of the head: I do not have to believe this yet.

Eyebrow: But what if it is true anyway?

Side of the eye: What if by allowing myself to feel this, it moves through me?

Under the eye: It does not stay stuck in me.

Under the nose: What if by feeling this, it really makes a difference?

Chin point: What if I will feel lighter after feeling it?

Collarbone: What if feeling fully is something I am intended to do?

Under the arm: What if this is necessary for me to feel better?

Top of the head: What if I am releasing stuck sadness right now?

Eyebrow: It is really just a feeling.

Side of the eye: It just feels potent because I am not used to accepting it.

Under the eye: What if it is the judgment I have carried around this that is really the issue?

Under the nose: If I accept my sadness and allow it, it moves through me.

Chin point: I like this idea.

Collarbone: It feels lighter, just feeling that it is okay.

Under the arm: If I feel my sadness, it will release and move through me.

Top of the head: I like this idea a lot.

Eyebrow: Of course, it is uncomfortable because I am not used to allowing it.

Side of the eye: What if it moves through me like it is intended to do?

Under the eye: I can learn to embrace my sadness more and more.

Under the nose: It is not something I have to be afraid of anymore.

Chin point: It is just a feeling, and it will move through me with my allowing of it.

Collarbone: It already feels a little better.

Under the arm: This sadness is not so bad.

Top of the head: I am open to healing more and more now.

Take a breath.

Rate how strong the feeling is now, from 0 (not strong at all) to 10 (extremely strong).

If the feeling is stronger, it means you have targeted the emotions. Go back and do the tapping sequence as often as you need to until you feel soothed, and these negative statements feel less true for you. This is a great indicator you are moving in the right direction.

How to Tap on Fear

Work your way through this entire segment, tapping on the point listed on the left as you say the corresponding statement out loud.

Karate chop: Even though I feel this fear, I choose to accept that I feel this way.

Karate chop: Even though I feel this fear and wish I did not, I choose to acknowledge that I feel this way.

Karate chop: Even though I feel this fear, it is not a feeling I like feeling, and I am judging myself for feeling this way.

Eyebrow: I am feeling this fear, and I do not like it.

Side of the eye: It is really uncomfortable.

Under the eye: I think I am really judging myself for this.

Under the nose: What if it is my judgment about my fear that is holding it in place?

Chin point: What if that is true?

Collarbone: Of course, I am judging myself.

Under the arm: I learned to treat myself the way I was treated.

Top of the head: I learned to judge myself the way I have been judged.

Eyebrow: What if judging myself is a habit that I have had for a long time?

Side of the eye: Fear is just a feeling.

Under the eye: I have learned to judge it as being wrong or bad.

Under the nose: I judge fear as a bad thing.

Chin point: What if it is not a bad thing?

Collarbone: It is just a feeling, and if it is allowed to move through me, it will.

Under the arm: What if it really is okay?

140

Top of the head: Where did I learn that fear is not okay?

Eyebrow: What if fear isn't good or bad...it is just fear?

Side of the eye: What if I learned a falsehood...

Under the eye: That I should eradicate fear, and I really don't need to?

Under the nose: What if the key to handling my fear is actually in accepting it first?

Chin point: What if fear is an indicator that I believe the bully in my brain?

Collarbone: What if I can see fear just this way?

Under the arm: What if by shifting the way I see fear, it doesn't have such a grip on me?

Top of the head: I like this idea more.

Eyebrow: I like the idea that fear can actually help me.

Side of the eye: What if fear reminds me I'm listening to the wrong voice?

Under the eye: I like this idea a lot.

Under the nose: Fear shows me where I believe what doesn't serve me well.

Chin point: It creates contrast, and if I can see it this way, it feels better to me.

Collarbone: I do not have to drown in fear if I can see it differently.

Under the arm: As I learn to release my self-judgment about fear...

Top of the head: It actually moves through me as it is intended to do.

Eyebrow: This idea feels lighter to me.

Side of the eye: Of course, I will feel fear in my life.

Under the eye: Everyone does, whether they admit it or not.

Under the Nose: What if I can take it off the list of Forbidden Emotions?

Chin point: What if I am starting to see fear differently, even now?

Collarbone: I like that I can get a better perspective on my emotions.

Under the arm: I have them for a reason.

Top of the head: What if the truth of them is that my emotions are my guides and they are actually really helpful to me as I see them in this way?

Take a breath.

Rate how strong the feeling is now, from 0 (not strong at all) to 10 (extremely strong).

If the feeling is stronger, it means you have targeted the emotions. Go back and do the

tapping sequence as often as you need to until you feel soothed, and these negative

statements feel less true for you. This is a great indicator you are moving in the right direction.

How to Tap on Joy

Work your way through this entire segment, tapping on the point listed on the left as you say the corresponding statement out loud.

Karate chop: Even though joy feels really good, sometimes I curb my joy so I do not hurt someone else who is feeling bad. I choose to accept myself anyway.

Karate chop: Even though sometimes I limit my feeling of joy around someone else, so they do not feel worse. I choose to acknowledge that this can happen for me.

Karate chop: Even though joy can be a Forbidden Emotion, I accept myself and my feelings now.

Eyebrow: Wow! This is eye-opening.

Side of the eye: I never saw how joy can be a problem, but it can.

Under the eye: It becomes problematic if I have to curb it.

Under the nose: I do not want others to feel bad.

Chin point: But it sucks, because things are going well for me, and I want to share that.

Collarbone: If I think my joy and good fortune might make someone else feel bad...

Under the arm: Then I curb it, and that actually sucks for me.

Top of the head: And I want to acknowledge this truth right now.

Eyebrow: Who knew joy could be a problem?

Side of the eye: But I see how it can be.

Under the eye: It is good to be aware of this.

Under the nose: I do not want someone else to feel bad, but I do not want to deny my joy.

Chin point: I have trouble with other emotions, so I would love to embrace my joy.

Collarbone: Joy feels great until I pinch it off.

Under the arm: It is good to be aware of this.

Top of the head: What if I cannot hide my joy enough to make it better for someone else?

Eyebrow: What if I am really not responsible for someone else's feelings?

Side of the eye: What if I actually do better for others when I embrace my joy?

Under the eye: What if I can learn to get better about this?

Under the nose: There does not have to be pressure to shift this. I can get there over time.

Chin point: I am a work in progress, and this is okay.

Collarbone: Just realizing that joy can be forbidden for me is a great start.

Under the arm: By knowing what I do not want, which is me curbing my joy...

Top of the head: I am getting clarity on what I do want, which is to embrace my joy.

Eyebrow: This clarity is helpful to me.

Side of the eye: My emotions are amazing.

Under the eye: They can guide me.

Under the nose: I can even get clearer over time about what I am feeling.

Chin point: I think I got trained not to feel too much of anything.

Collarbone: What if I am learning to feel fully and embrace my amazing emotions?

Under the arm: I came into this world with emotions...

Top of the head: So, they must be there for a reason.

Eyebrow: I like the idea that all of my emotions are here to help me.

Side of the eye: I like the idea that I can feel all of them more fully.

Under the eye: I like the idea that as I allow myself joy in all circumstances...

Under the nose: I am learning to appreciate all that my emotions have to say to me.

Chin point: Joy is just another emotion I can learn to feel fully.

Collarbone: My emotions are amazing.

Under the arm: As I learn to embrace my joy, I am learning to love myself more and more.

Top of the head: And more good will continue to come.

Take a breath.

Rate how strong the feeling is now, from 0 (not strong at all) to 10 (extremely strong).

If the feeling is stronger, it means you have targeted the emotions. Go back and do the tapping sequence as often as you need to until you feel soothed, and these negative statements feel less true for you. This is a great indicator you are moving in the right direction.

How to Tap on Frustration

Work your way through this entire segment, tapping on the point listed on the left as you say the corresponding statement out loud.

Karate chop: Even though I am really frustrated, I choose to accept myself anyway.

Karate chop: Even though I feel really frustrated, I choose to acknowledge I feel this way.

Karate chop: Even though I feel really, really frustrated, and I do not like it at all, I choose to accept myself anyway.

Eyebrow: All of this frustration.

Side of the eye: I feel it in my body.

Under the eye: I am really frustrated.

Under the nose: It really has a grip on me.

Chin point: What if I am judging myself for feeling this way?

Collarbone: What if it is the judgment that is keeping this in place?

Under the arm: What if I have a right to feel frustrated?

Top of the head: It is a frustrating situation.

Eyebrow: What if it is normal to feel frustrated under these circumstances?

Side of the eye: It is a frustrating circumstance.

Under the eye: My frustration is telling me something.

Under the nose: My frustration is an indicator.

Chin point: It is just another emotion that is in me for a reason.

Collarbone: My frustration tells me what is happening for me.

Under the arm: And that is a good thing if I can see it that way.

Top of the head: It is just an emotional indicator.

Eyebrow: There's nothing wrong with me feeling this way.

Side of the eye: It is an emotion that I have that is there for a reason.

Under the eye: There's nothing wrong with frustration.

Under the nose: It is one of the amazing emotions that I came into this life with.

Chin point: What if I can learn to welcome my feelings more and more?

Collarbone: As I allow for frustration, it is allowed to move through me.

Under the arm: That is what it is intended to do.

Top of the head: And when it is allowed to move through me, I am learning how emotions

work for me.

Eyebrow: I am really frustrated, but that is okay.

Side of the eye: I am really frustrated, and I am allowing it.

Under the eye: I am frustrated, and it is just an emotion.

Under the nose: My frustration is indicating something's off for me.

Chin point: My emotions are working.

Collarbone: My emotions are meant to be in me.

Under the arm: There's nothing bad or wrong with any emotion.

Top of the head: It is when I suppress them that my actions of suppressing them can feel bad to me.

Eyebrow: What if by feeling them, I learn to express myself more healthfully?

Side of the eye: What if I can acknowledge and truly feel my feelings, and what if this helps me?

Under the eye: I can begin to express myself in the best way.

Under the nose: I like this idea very much.

Chin point: As I begin to feel my feelings more fully, I am better able to express myself...

Collarbone: In a healthier way.

Under the arm: I like this idea a lot.

Top of the head: And what if I am starting to do that right now?

Take a breath.

Rate how strong the feeling is now, from 0 (not strong at all) to 10 (extremely strong).

If the feeling is stronger, it means you have targeted the emotions. Go back and do the tapping sequence as often as you need to until you feel soothed, and these negative statements feel less true for you. This is a great indicator you are moving in the right direction.

(Disclaimer: Please note, the f-word is used in this script. Honor yourself and do what feels best for you.)

How to Tap on Shame

Shame is often called the silent killer of our spirit. As Janice Berger says in her book, *Emotional Fitness.*

> "Shame is a silent killer because it prevents us from revealing to the world who we really are. When we hold onto our shame as an adult it can be totally debilitating. Like worthlessness, shame becomes a devastating defense because it keeps us stuck...We become shame-bound if it was unacceptable for us to express them."

Let's begin to unravel shame.

Karate chop: Even though I have feelings of shame that I learned to reject, using any other emotion to cover shame up, I choose to accept myself anyway.

Karate chop: Even though I really avoid feeling shame, I choose to acknowledge this now.

Karate chop: Even though I do not want to feel shame because I learned to reject it from those around me, I do not like it at all, and I want to accept myself anyway.

Eyebrow: I feel so ashamed.

Side of the Eye: I have a belief that I should feel ashamed.

Under the eye: I do not want to feel shame because it feels overwhelming.

Under the nose: I know I carry shame, but I do not want this.

149

Chin point: I am afraid of this shame.

Collarbone: It feels terrible.

Under the arm: I may have no idea how to release this shame.

Top of the head: What if I am starting to right now?

Eyebrow: I do not want to hear myself about my shame.

Side of the eye: This sucks.

Under the eye: I have spent most of my life avoiding shame.

Under the Nose: What if I can learn to stay present with myself and the feeling of shame?

Chin point: No way!

Collarbone: No way!

Under the arm: I refuse to feel this shame.

Top of the head: This is not going to help me.

Eyebrow: It just debilitates me.

Side of the eye: This will not happen.

Under the eye: I say, "fuck you," to this shame.

Under the nose: This is not going to help me.

Chin point: I do not see the point.

Collarbone: I refuse to feel this, and no one can make me.

Under the arm: Fuck it.

Top of the head: Fuck this shame.

Eyebrow: What is the point?

Side of the eye: It is not going to change anything.

Under the eye: It may be too soon to believe this, but what if it really can help?

Under the nose: Bullshit.

Chin point: I refuse to believe this.

Collarbone: I refuse to be that vulnerable.

Under the arm: It is dangerous and unsafe to feel shame.

Top of the head: No way!

Eyebrow: What if right now I don't have to feel shame?

Side of the eye: What if I don't ever have to feel the shame?

Under the eye: You got that right!

Under the Nose: What if I can just acknowledge the possibility that I carry shame?

Chin point: What if there's actually nothing wrong with me for carrying shame?

Collarbone: What if this very belief has been holding it in place?

Under the arm: The belief that shame is bad or forbidden.

Top of the head: What if I can be open to the idea that shame is not bad or forbidden?

Eyebrow: What if by just creating a tiny little opening here in my beliefs, that is enough?

Side of the eye: What if shame is just another emotion that I learned to reject and deny?

Under the eye: What if I may have nothing to be ashamed of? Could this be possible?

Under the Nose: What if I learned to believe lies...that feel like truths?

Chin point: What if one of those lies is that I should feel ashamed?

Collarbone: I kinda like this idea, whether I believe it yet or not.

Under the arm: What if I had to hide my feelings as a child, but I don't have to hide them now?

Top of the head: What if shame is not as big of a deal as I learned it was?

Eyebrow: What?

Side of the eye: What if it doesn't have to be so debilitating?

Under the eye: What if there's an upside to shame?

Under the nose: What if it lets me know I need to rethink something?

Chin point: What if it really could be okay?

Collarbone: What if shame doesn't have to be this hideous monster at all?

Under the arm: What if I can be open to this idea, just a little bit?

Top of the head: What if I can just entertain this possibility?

Eyebrow: I do not have to decide about this today.

Side of the eye: What if there's some truth in all of this?

Under the eye: What if I can consider this and see what comes?

Under the nose: What if considering this helps me to lighten up about shame?

Chin point: I like this idea a lot.

Collarbone: I like the idea of putting less pressure on myself around shame.

Under the arm: What if this is enough for now?

Top of the head: What if accepting shame as another emotion is a start?

Take a breath.

Rate how strong the feeling is now, from 0 (not strong at all) to 10 (extremely strong).

If the feeling is stronger, it means you have targeted the emotions. Go back and do the tapping sequence as often as you need to until you feel soothed, and these negative statements feel less true for you. This is a great indicator you are moving in the right direction.

How to Tap on Guilt

Karate chop: Even though I feel guilt, and I do not like it at all, I choose to acknowledge that I feel this way.

Karate chop: Even though I feel guilt and wish I did not, I choose to acknowledge myself anyway now.

Karate chop: Even though I can really feel guilt, it is not a feeling I like at all, because I know it holds me back.

Eyebrow: I am feeling this guilt, and I do not like it.

Side of the eye: It is really uncomfortable.

Under the eye: I think I am really judging myself for this.

153

Under the nose: What if it is my judgment about my guilt that is holding it in place?

Chin point: What if that is true?

Collarbone: Of course, I am judging myself.

Under the arm: I learned to treat myself the way I was treated.

Top of the head: I learned to judge myself the way I have been judged.

Eyebrow: What if judging myself is a habit that I have had for a long time?

Side of the eye: Guilt is a feeling I am awfully familiar with.

Under the eye: I have learned to keep myself in line using guilt to do it.

Under the nose: What if this stuck guilt no longer serves me well at all?

Chin point: What if guilt holds me back now?

Collarbone: Guilt is just another feeling, and if it is allowed to move through me, it will.

Under the arm: What if it really is okay to release this guilt?

Top of the head: What if it is time to let it go?

Eyebrow: What if I learned to assign blame to myself every time I feel guilty?

Side of the eye: What if I no longer need to hold myself hostage using guilt?

Under the eye: What if this guilt I have carried has never even been mine?

154

Under the nose: What if it is okay to let this guilt drift away?

Chin point: What if guilt is good when it helps me to redirect myself in a good way?

Collarbone: But the guilt I have been carrying has been debilitating, and that is not good for me.

Under the arm: What if, by making it okay to release the guilt, I shift my life for the better?

Top of the head: I like this idea a lot, even if I am not convinced of this yet.

Eyebrow: I like the idea that it is time to let go of this guilt.

Side of the eye: I like the idea that this could be possible.

Under the eye: I like that I am at least exploring releasing guilt.

Under the nose: I like that this could be a possibility for me.

Chin point: I am just exploring a possibility.

Collarbone: I do not have to let it go yet if part of me does not feel safe doing so.

Under the arm: And as I learn to release even a little guilt, it just may help.

Top of the head: I like the idea that I no longer have to hold myself hostage to guilt.

Eyebrow: This idea feels lighter to me.

Side of the eye: Of course, I will feel guilt in my life.

Under the eye: Everyone does, whether they admit it or not.

Under the Nose: What if I can take it off the list of Forbidden Emotions?

Chin point: What if I am starting to see guilt differently, even now?

Collarbone: I like that I can get a better perspective about guilt.

Under the arm: I like that guilt can be felt and released, as it is meant to be.

Top of the head: What if the truth about guilt is that it is another one of my emotions that can guide me and help me?

Take a breath.

Rate how strong the feeling is now, from 0 (not strong at all) to 10 (extremely strong).

If the feeling is stronger, it means you have targeted the emotions. Go back and do the tapping sequence as often as you need to until you feel soothed, and these negative statements feel less true for you. This is a great indicator you are moving in the right direction.

Note on These Tapping Scripts

These scripts are intended to assist you in getting in touch with what your forbidden emotions are. Go back and use them as often as you need to uncover emotions off limits to you.

The more familiar you get with the emotions that feel off-limits for you, the more your awareness helps you to catch yourself "should"ing on your feelings. When you find this, you are better able to begin to process your emotions and thus release them.

Now let's move on and take this a step deeper by learning a highly effective way to release Forbidden Emotions.

Chapter Summary

Learning the Basics of Tapping is the most effective way I know to uncover and safely discharge forbidden emotions. It allows you to access the unconscious programming that's been activated throughout your life.

It's a simple, slightly strange, yet highly effective technique that's literally at your fingertips that you can use daily as needed. If you follow the five steps to effective tapping on a target, this will become second nature to you.

I believe you'll realize this truly has the power to soothe your stress. If done consistently, you'll recognize the cumulative effect. You'll want to use it more to help you process through emotions any time you need to.

You'll no longer feel afraid of any emotion. This is a huge benefit because it allows you the confidence to manage your emotional life more effectively, which helps your self-confidence grow.

Rant Tapping

(AKA "Fuck You" Tapping)

Disclaimer:
Before you proceed, know this chapter uses several expletives. If you are sensitive to words considered profane, bypass this chapter. But if you can keep an open mind to the purpose of using these words, then you might find some internal liberation in this chapter. Either way, please take responsibility for yourself and make the choice you feel is most honorable to you.

There are more tapping sequences in this chapter, so know that powerful emotions can surface, and this shows that we have targeted an emotion. Please take responsibility for yourself and keep tapping until you feel soothed. Always consult your therapist or medical doctor before going through these exercises.

Something for you to consider in deciding if you will read this chapter. Tapping worked well in my, and my clients' lives. Allow yourself the full expression of forbidden thoughts, and you will find liberation on the other side.

You find this because tapping can help you release and neutralize these forbidden thoughts, experiences, and emotions within you anyway. You may have learned these thoughts, experiences, and emotions are inappropriate to express, but what if you can do this in a safe, private, and effective way? One possibility is you experience true emotional freedom, even genuine compassion, forgiveness, and peace, without having to "try" to find compassion or "try" to forgive someone. Compassion and forgiveness are often natural by-products of feeling fully and expressing and thus releasing what has been seen as forbidden.

The process behind Rant Tapping is that you rant out your thoughts while tapping. This is usually when you are angry. While tapping through the points, you rant out your feelings.

Rant tapping is a style of tapping I did not create. I was taught it when I was getting my EFT Certification. I have found it to be effective with Forbidden Emotions. No one I trained with called Rant tapping "fuck you" tapping, but it is a term I used the more I worked with Rant Tapping with clients.

I use the term "fuck you" tapping with Rant Tapping. I came to call it "fuck you" tapping because of what would happen during sessions with clients.

When I work with clients upset with someone, I ask them:
"If you could say anything to this person... I mean anything... what would you say?"

Before they begin, I tell clients to put being appropriate on the shelf for now. They can pick that back up after this, but when working with their anger, I ask them not to worry about propriety. It opens a doorway for liberation when you get to the other side of releasing anger or rage.

Nine times out of ten, when I ask my clients what they would say to someone who upset them, they say:

"I'd say 'fuck you' to them."

There can be variations of this, most of which add a gender-specific swear word, if you catch my drift.

159

I tell them to go on and rant tap, but to be sure they are tapping the entire time and letting this person have it. This is their chance to let out all the suppressed emotions. They get to say to this person anything and everything they have ever wanted to say to them, they stopped themselves from saying.

I encourage clients by reassuring them that with me is a safe place to do this; the person they are upset with will never hear their words. This is the healthiest way to release pent-up anger, frustration, hurt, sadness, and more. Whatever surfaces is good and necessary.

The beauty of this process is how it feels after. When you have a healthy, safe way to unearth and release your Forbidden Emotions as it relates to someone who upsets you, you do not hurt them by lashing out. You do not hurt yourself by burying it and causing turmoil in your body.

Set Yourself Free

These are the words virtually all my clients have said after they're done rant tapping: "I feel liberated."

This was true for me. When I have done this in my life, I have come out the other side feeling liberated. Freed from the ties that have bound me.

A huge upside is that when you free yourself in this way, you will find you behave differently around this person. It frees you from acting out with them in ways that chip away at your self-esteem.

As an example. Say there's someone in your life who hurt you deeply, and every time you have tried to talk to them, it just seems to feel worse.

They cannot meet you halfway or even a fraction of the way. You harbor an even bigger resentment and feelings of how unfair this all is.

When you allow yourself—privately or helped by a seasoned practitioner—to say everything you would love to say to them, no matter how inappropriate, you free yourself from your intense feelings toward them.

The benefit is you can end up in a place where you no longer need them to admit or help you resolve anything. You've resolved it within yourself. This is the only true power and freedom we have.

You have given yourself your full-throttle truth safely, and you liberate yourself. This is the only true freedom we ever have. Freeing ourselves from within.

The beauty of using this method to release potent emotions is the person you're upset with will often own their part in things or even apologize. This happens because you've released the stuck emotional energy.

When you do this, you will find you are no longer attached to needing them to either own their part or apologize, but you will get it anyway.

You are emotionally free. I call this a win-win. I had one client do this about a sibling she felt was out to destroy her. After our first Rant Tapping session, her sister's lawyer contacted her with some disturbing news, and she laughed. That is the power of Rant Tapping.

She admits to still getting triggered, and I do too, but it gets better the more you do it.

You still have a human experience, and part of the human condition is that you get triggered by the events and people in your life. When you know you have an effective technique that can help to ease the anger, rage, or fury you feel, it feels less overwhelming and less like you will never stop feeling this way. When you make a practice of tapping, over time, it has a cumulative effect that changes you. You will notice more times where you may have gotten triggered in the past, but now you are not. There's a progression to this over time where you become more aware of your own improvement. This lets you know that you are changing.

I have yet to see someone use Rant Tapping and not change for the better. Especially if they keep using it when needed.

Rant tapping is the most powerful tapping technique I have found when dealing with Forbidden Emotions. It gives you a way to release them, with no one being hurt. You are not walking up to this person and spewing all of your anger at them. You are doing it on your own or with a professional in a private space.

You realize there are not any worthless emotions. If an emotion is felt through to its completion, we release it. When trying to tell ourselves we should not feel something we felt, the behaviors we might display as a result can be problematic, embarrassing, and potentially deadly in the worst cases.

In her book, *"Crazy Time: Surviving Divorce and Building a New Life,"* Abigail Trafford talks about how we can be a little crazy when going through a divorce.

"Most people go a little crazy when their marriage cracks open. You are rarely prepared for the practical or emotional turmoil that lies ahead. You swing between euphoria, violent rage, and depression. You may search frenetically for a new mate or you go the other way and withdraw from people and not answer the phone. Health statistics tell you that you are prone to getting sick and having car accidents. Reports of triangle assaults and murders of estranged spouses make regular newspaper headlines. In the dark hours of loneliness, you think about suicide. At some point, almost everyone coming out of a marriage mutters to what was once the other half 'I could kill you.'

If everyone going through a potent emotional experience could use Rant Tapping, it would shorten the emotional learning curve and be a lot more manageable. It does not suppress their emotions; it encourages them to surface. The tapping allows the procession of the emotions. The natural by-product of this, which brings a great upside, is that it releases the emotions from your nervous system. Once released, there's no need for them to leak out in destructive behaviors.

Think of it this way: you are releasing, not building up, stuck emotions.

It encourages you to "get it all out" and to "be brutally honest." Getting the emotions out and being brutally honest in a private, safe, supported environment, without spewing all your brutal honesty out on the person, creates true liberation. You free the most important person in your life—you—from the emotional ties that have bound you up. The other part of this is that you free the other person. This allows you to deal with this person from a healthier vantage point, which elevates your emotional fitness. As a by-product of this, your self-esteem increases.

When I work with clients in this way, I always ask their permission to use Rant Tapping. I understand most of us have been programmed to have Forbidden Emotions. Allowing ourselves to feel fully and to speak our truth can feel daunting.

When this happens, I often need to tap on guilt with clients first. This helps to create an openness, allowing them to acknowledge and then say what has been rumbling around inside them toward someone.

Once we have created an opening by releasing some guilt, they are more likely to be brutally honest about their feelings and what they would like to say to someone. We tap while allowing all the Forbidden Emotions to surface through the forbidden words. On the other side of this is liberation.

Unleash Your Inner Ability to Create Whatever You Want

When you allow yourself the space to release the thoughts and feelings attached to these emotions that have felt off-limits to you, you release negativity. This allows who you are to come shining through. That is why you notice that without trying, you become more positive.

I use this analogy: The sun is always in the sky somewhere. It is always there. Sometimes clouds move in and block it from view, but it is still always there. Releasing emotional blocks is like the clouds moving out so you can see the sun shining. This is the truth of you.

You came into this life experience loaded with all the amenities. Along the way, clouds moved in, emotional blocks or limiting beliefs. These blocked you from remembering the truth of you: that you are an infinite being with the innate ability to lead a fulfilling life. This happens when you free yourself from the emotional blocks that have been in the way. As you do so, inspired thoughts can come into your conscious awareness. You gain access to take inspired action as you recognize it. Your life gets better because you connect back in with the infinite being you are.

The Best Time to Use Rant Tapping

The best time to use Rant Tapping is when you have or have had strong anger or rage about a person, place, or circumstance. I say "have or have had" because we can bury the anger and rage. Tapping is most effective when the emotions are present. Therefore, I ask clients the question. "If you could say anything to this person, anything at all, what would you say?" This is a way to get in touch with suppressed emotions. If a client is already experiencing a strong emotion, then we start Rant Tapping.

Sometimes clients will ask me to help start them, and then they take over and rant away while tapping. Sometimes their pump is primed, and they rant away on their own while tapping.

Tapping while ranting is particularly important. It will help you move the energy through you more quickly by soothing your nervous system and changing your physiology.

Rant tapping is the technique I used with my client I discussed before, diagnosed with a benign, inoperable brain tumor. She ranted away all the suppressed emotion she had toward the people in her life with whom she was angry. She is convinced this is the reason her tumor shrunk. She told her doctor it is the only thing she had done out of the ordinary.

165

In my life, when I started tapping and got honest with myself, what I felt toward my parents was hatred. The statement I said out loud to myself one day was, "I hate them."

I took photos of my parents, looked at these photos, and spent close to forty-five minutes ranting. All the injustices my sisters and I experienced at the hands of our parents came out. I was raging while I tapped. Once I moved through the anger, I felt deep sadness, and I wept. I trusted the tapping and kept tapping on each emotion that surfaced, and before I knew it, I was laughing.

I said silly things to them in my tapping. I felt so much lighter. It releases all the heaviness I lugged around like a ball and chain, keeping me emotionally imprisoned. It was a transformational experience.

My parents were deceased for a few years, so I was not saying this to them in person. The amazing upside is that I felt free. I also believe I set them free.

I said the statement, "My parents did the best they could," and I noticed I finally felt congruent with this statement. It was true for me now. I would have choked on this statement and felt like it was not true, all while shoving down and suppressing what I felt: pissed, robbed, ripped off, and even betrayed. As I write this, I believe they did the best they could. I also understand they were buried in their own Forbidden Emotions.

Please do not feel like you need to jump right into telling yourself, *"My parents did the best they could."* Without going through the Rant Tapping—releasing all the stuck emotions—it does not serve you. You will know when you are free because when you say it out loud, you will believe that they did the best they could. You will feel it emotionally, not intellectually.

I say it this way: what happened with my parents happened. Since they are no longer here in physical form, I have no new experiences to deal with.

If some memory of my past with them surfaces, I do not feel the same angst and anger I did before. I tap on what comes up, and it seems to move on.

My first Rant Tapping cleared a pathway to forgiveness for me. I am not suggesting that I need not attend to any memories that surface about them, because I do, but somehow it is different now. The compassion I have for them now is always there, even when some potent memories surface.

When dealing with people in your life who are still alive, Rant Tapping can be your new best friend. It will allow you to release as you need to so that when you have to deal with them, you will notice you can better do so.

When working with clients, the actual rant or "fuck you" tapping sequences are often very dynamic. They often release a lot of anger and rage.

If you are new to this tapping, find a seasoned professional so they can help to facilitate it for you if you are leery of this. Many of my clients have taken to this form of tapping like a duck to water. Not everyone needs to do this tapping, but I find many people do not realize at first just how much anger they have suppressed.

How to Tell If You Need Rant Tapping?

One way to know you need to rant tap is if you notice your anger, in an innocuous situation, feels over-the-top. This is often an indicator of suppressed emotion.

A client I worked with once experienced anger as her primary Forbidden Emotion. I asked her the question I recommended: *"If you could say anything to your parents, what would you say?"* I encouraged her to leave being appropriate at the door.

She felt like she should not hate them, which showed that she felt anger. Her face would contort as a flash of anger would surface, and she would make excuses for the abusive behavior directed at her. She would say she knows they had it rough, too.

Now, this is always the case. The saying "hurt people hurt people" is true, but when you use statements of truth to block you from feeling fully then you reach for a box of donuts, down too much alcohol, or run to a casino and blow money you don't have, aren't you hurting you? Isn't that a problem for you?

My client was desperate to lose about 40 pounds of excess weight. Still, it was clear she could not even attempt that goal before doing the prep work. She needed to allow herself to share how she felt about her parents during a private session they would not be privy to.

The resistance a client has to the truth is often equal to the suppression that has occurred around emotions for them.

When your emotions are not validated, no matter what they are, you suppress them. When invalidated every time you express your emotions, you suppress them. If you are lamenting about your car breaking down, and money for repairs and some well-meaning person says, "Look on the bright side; Joe down the street just lost his wife," more suppression occurs.

I do not care if someone ate your leftovers, or you got a stain on your favorite shirt; your emotions are valid to you.

Whenever you, or someone else, compares your circumstances to others to make you "feel better," you suppress emotions.

When you learn to allow yourself to feel fully, you process your emotions through to their completion, and not at the expense of someone else, especially yourself. By that, I mean, we do not intend Rant Tapping to be a bully pulpit to bully someone else.

Be "brutally honest" in your Rant Tapping sessions when you are ready to. Still, it is not at all intended as an excuse for bad behavior. I say this because many of my clients have encountered someone being "brutally honest" to their faces under the guise of "just being honest." I call bullshit on this. Be honest privately to yourself or with a skilled EFT practitioner or therapist where no one gets hurt. You get to release privately, which is the healthiest, most effective way to use this technique. I have never suggested that anyone go spew their anger to someone.

Rant Tapping Scripts

For the rest of this chapter, I will share a sequence of tapping scripts to help you experience the transformative power of Rant Tapping.

Tapping Sequence #1: Attending to Guilt about Rant Tapping

I find guilt is often the first thing we need to deal with before someone will allow themselves to go for it using Rant Tapping to clear emotions. Here are the steps that will reveal if your guilt needs tapping first:

Think about someone you feel has wronged you. Someone who has never apologized for what they did.

What feeling is attached to this?

Rate how strong the feeling is, from 0 (not strong at all) to 10 (extremely strong).

Notice: if you feel angry, do you notice guilt about feeling this way? If you do, then use the first sequence below. If you do not feel guilt, go to Tapping Sequence #2.

If you feel guilty about being angry with this person, then we want to attend to that first.

169

When using this first sequence, edit the words as you need to. If something pops up in your head, that feels more accurate than what the script says, say what is truer for you instead.

This will help you target what is happening to you. Your brain will feed you what fits you best. If this resonates, use it as is.

Karate chop:

Even though I am furious with _____, I do not feel right about expressing my anger. Anger is dangerous. It is not good to feel too much. I acknowledge I feel this way.

Even though I am furious with _____, it is hard for me to say this because I know they have their issues too. I acknowledge my feelings now.

Even though I am furious with _____, I do not want to feel this way. Anger is not something I am comfortable feeling. I have seen a lot of bad things that too much anger causes. I accept myself and my feelings now.

Eyebrow: Anger is not okay.

Side of the eye: It is wrong and even worse to feel it.

Under the eye: Maybe it is okay to feel it a little.

Under the nose: But it is definitely not good to feel too much of it.

Chin point: It is destructive.

Collarbone: I do not want to be like them anyway.

Under the arm: I want to be the bigger person.

Top of the head: I should be the bigger person.

170

Eyebrow: This is the best way to be.

Side of the eye: If I allow myself to be furious, I will be just like them.

Under the eye: I want to be better than that.

Under the nose: What if maybe I am burying my anger?

Chin point: What if there's nothing wrong with feeling the anger itself?

Collarbone: It is just an emotion.

Under the arm: What if it is better for me to feel it fully?

Top of the head: What if nobody has to witness it but me and maybe someone that is helping me with it?

Eyebrow: What if by dealing with my anger this way, I release it from my energy system?

Side of the eye: What if by releasing it, I can much better deal with this person?

Under the eye: What if by allowing myself to free myself from my anger...

Under the nose: I actually give myself a gift.

Chin point: I was born with a full palette of emotions.

Collarbone: What if there isn't a good or bad emotion?

Under the arm: What if there are negative and positive emotions, but they are not good or bad?

Top of the head: I mean, why do I have these emotions?

Eyebrow: What if my emotions guide me if I can see them that way?

Side of the eye: What if my anger is just a great indicator for me?

171

Under the eye: What if my anger lets me know there's something wrong within myself, and there's nothing wrong with this?

Under the nose: What if by allowing myself to feel my anger...

Chin point: I no longer bury it.

Collarbone: What if by feeling it fully, I release it?

Under the arm: What if it does what all emotions do?

Top of the head: It moves through me much more quickly.

Eyebrow: What if by feeling all of my feelings fully safely...

Side of the eye: I become more emotionally fit...

Under the eye: More emotionally intelligent.

Under the nose: And what if this is the best thing for me?

Chin point: I need not say anything to their face when I am angry.

Collarbone: What if I can do it in a safe, private space?

Under the arm: So I can feel my anger through to its completion.

Top of the head: And what if once I do this...

Eyebrow: It leaves my energy system.

Side of the eye: And what if from this place, I can better handle myself...

Under the eye: Because I am honoring all of me and my emotions.

Under the nose: I came into this life installed with a full range of emotions.

Chin point: An amazing palette of emotions that can help me.

Collarbone: As I learn to accept all of my emotions...

Under the arm: I stop judging any of them as forbidden or off-limits...

Top of the head: And by doing so....

Eyebrow: I set myself free.

Side of the eye: Over time...I can much better feel fully at any moment.

Under the eye: The upside of this is that I can far better manage myself.

Under the nose: Feelings are just feelings.

Chin point: And if I learn to feel them fully...

Collarbone: They release on their own.

Under the arm: When released in this way...

Top of the head: They do not come up at the most inopportune time anymore.

Eyebrow: And what if this is better for me?

Side of the eye: And better for everyone involved.

Under the eye: I like this idea a lot.

Under the nose: This feels lighter to see it this way.

Chin point: What if by honoring my feelings, no matter what they are...

Collarbone: I will notice I feel better and better.

Under the arm: What if I see my emotions as indicators of where I am, and this helps me learn not to judge myself for my emotions?

173

Top of the head: What if I can try it and see what happens?

Take a breath.

That round is to acknowledge guilt that may surface, so you can clear it first and become better able to get the maximum benefit out of the following round.

Rate how strong the guilt is now from 0 (not strong at all) to 10 (extremely strong).

If it is the same—or gone higher—do this round as often as you need until the guilt is at two or below. If you cannot land on a number, then notice if you feel less attached to the guilt.

Once you feel ready for the next round, we will deal with anger.

Tapping Sequence #2: Rant Tapping

Let's move on to Rant Tapping. Begin with these steps:

Think about someone you feel has wronged you. Someone who never apologized for what they did.

What feeling is attached to this?

Rate how strong the feeling is from 0 (not strong at all) to 10 (extremely strong).

Now use the following script and edit it as you need to. If something pops up in your head that feels more accurate than what the script says, then say what is truer for you instead. This will help you target what is happening for you. You'll know if you need to change the words because they will pop into your head while tapping.

We go right to the eyebrow with Rant Tapping and start with the unedited truth.

Eyebrow: I am so pissed about this.

Side of the eye: God, I am angry.

Under the eye: What the hell?

Under the nose: Are you kidding me?

Chin point: How could they do that?

Collarbone: And not apologize.

Under the arm: I always apologize when I feel I am wrong.

Top of the head: Why can't they ever apologize?

Eyebrow: I mean, what the fuck.

Side of the eye: This is ridiculous.

Under the eye: Why is it so hard for them to apologize? I do it, even when I do not want to.

Under the nose: It would make things so much better.

Chin point: What a fucking asshole.

Collarbone: Gaaaaaawwww!

Under the arm: What were they thinking?

Top of the head: How can they be that unreasonable?

Eyebrow: This is so infuriating.

Side of the eye: I just do not get it.

Under the eye: It makes me so upset.

Under the nose: What the hell?

Chin point: This is so unfair.

Collarbone: I just do not get it.

Under the arm: I will never understand them.

175

Top of the head: How do people do that?

Eyebrow: Say hurtful crap and then never think to say they are sorry.

Side of the eye: I will never understand this.

Under the eye: I feel like I cannot get over this unless they apologize.

Under the nose: They refuse to see my side of things.

Chin point: What a fucking jerk.

Collarbone: I mean, who does that?

Under the arm: Who says mean shit and never takes ownership?

Top of the head: The worst part is that they actually think it is my fault.

Eyebrow: What the fuck!

Side of the eye: This is so infuriating.

Under the eye: I am so pissed.

Under the nose: I apologized, and now they are acting all smug.

Chin point: This makes me feel even worse.

Collarbone: What the hell is wrong with me that I apologized to them?

Under the arm: I feel so pathetic.

Top of the head: I am pathetic.

Eyebrow: When will I ever learn?

Side of the eye: That stupid smug look on their face.

Under the eye: It's like they know they have won.

Under the nose: They got me to apologize and take the blame.

Chin point: I am so fucking mad I did that.

Collarbone: I feel like such a wimp.

Under the arm: I am a wimp.

Top of the head: I am right to judge myself.

Eyebrow: What a fucking joke.

Side of the eye: I fucking apologized.

Under the eye: I have done this so often.

Under the nose: Someone treats me like shit...

Chin point: And I fucking apologize.

Collarbone: They are such a fucking asshole.

Under the arm: They never take ownership.

Top of the head: I want to scream; I am so mad.

Eyebrow: They suck.

Side of the eye: This is such bullshit.

Under the eye: I cannot believe I am back here again.

Under the nose: I am so fucking pissed.

Chin point: I am beyond pissed.

Collarbone: I want to scream. (Scream if you need to.)

Under the arm: I hate this shit.

Top of the Head: I want to tell them to fuck off.

Eyebrow: I have a right to feel this way.

Side of the Eye: They are so fucking infuriating.

Under the Eye: I can't believe how angry I feel.

Under the Nose: What if I actually own my anger right now?

Chin Point: What if I can keep letting myself feel this angry and tap my way through it?

Collarbone: What if this feels so potent because I'm allowing this anger up and out?

Under the arm: What if this is a good thing?

Top of the head: What if by allowing this anger, I also allow it to move on when I'm ready?

Eyebrow: I have been stuffing my anger for way too long.

Side of the eye: What if by owning this and finally allowing myself my feelings...

Under the eye: I can get to the other side of this?

Under the nose: I am so tired of telling myself I should not feel anger.

Chin point: I am so tired of telling myself that any of my emotions are off-limits.

Collarbone: What if, over time, I can take a step back?

Under the arm: What if this is an excellent place to start?

Top of the head: With owning my own feelings and seeing what comes from this.

Take a breath.

Rate how strong the feeling is now from 0 (not strong at all) to 10 (extremely strong).

If the feeling is stronger, it means you have targeted the emotions. Go back and do the tapping sequence as often as you need. Once you feel soothed, and the unedited statements feel less true for you and the more positive, bridging statements feel more true. This is a great indicator you are moving in the right direction.

Once you feel soothed and your number is two or below, go to the next round.

Tapping Sequence #3: Bridging Round to the Positive

Eyebrow: Wow! I see that I am furious at myself.

Side of the eye: The person I have judged the most is me.

Under the eye: I am judging them too, and that is okay.

Under the nose: I am hurt, so I am judging them for what they did.

Chin point: What if I really need to attend to my harsh judgment of myself?

Collarbone: What if this is the place to start?

Under the arm: I may feel adamant I deserve to judge myself, but...

Top of the head: What if I can be just a little open to healing this?

Eyebrow: It hurts to judge myself.

Side of the eye: To call myself names.

Under the eye: To say mean things to myself.

179

Under the nose: Whoa! What if their judgment of me actually mirrors my internal judgment of myself? Dammit. What if this is true?

Chin point: I do not want to admit that, and that is okay.

Collarbone: But what if, at least on some level, this is true?

Under the arm: What if I can be open to shifting this?

Top of the head: I learned to treat myself the way they treated me.

Eyebrow: If I think about it, this is true.

Side of the eye: This is a unique way of seeing things.

Under the eye: I learned to treat myself the way they treated me.

Under the nose: So, what if this person is mirroring this judgment to me?

Chin point: I need not like them.

Collarbone: I need not like what they have done or said.

Under the arm: Not at all.

Top of the head: But what if I can be even a little open to what I can learn here?

Eyebrow: What if I am getting a picture of how I have been treating myself?

Side of the eye: What if I can learn to be a little nicer to myself?

Under the eye: I may have no clue how to do this yet, but what if I can learn over time?

Under the nose: What if by learning to be kinder to me...

Chin point: This is a big key to creating change for me?

Collarbone: What if by making this a priority...

Under the arm: I change what happens in my life?

Top of the head: What if it starts with me?

Eyebrow: What if by learning to be nicer to me...

Side of the eye: I attract people nicer to me?

Under the eye: What if it is possible that even the people in my life...

Under the nose: Who are not so nice to me, end up being nicer...

Chin point: Because I am nicer to myself.

Collarbone: What if this is true?

Under the arm: I need not believe this yet.

Top of the head: But what if I can be open to this idea?

Eyebrow: This is the only place I have any power to change.

Side of the eye: God knows I have tried to get others to change.

Under the eye: So far, I have been unsuccessful at that.

Under the nose: If I think about it...

Chin point: I feel powerless when I try to get someone else to change.

Collarbone: It is futile.

Under the arm: What if it starts with me?

Top of the head: By shifting the focus to myself...

Eyebrow: I have power here.

Side of the eye: It might take me a while.

181

Under the eye: I have to unlearn a lot of things I have learned.

Under the Nose: That have kept me feeling disempowered.

Chin point: What if I can cut myself some slack?

Collarbone: What if I will always be a work in progress?

Under the arm: What if I can embrace this concept?

Top of the head: What if this could take some pressure off?

Eyebrow: I like this idea, even if I do not believe it yet.

Side of the eye: There's something about it that feels true on some level.

Under the eye: At least this is a start.

Under the Nose: What if the outcome of shifting myself is that I attract more of the things I desire?

Chin point: I like this idea a lot.

Collarbone: I enjoy putting pressure on myself.

Under the arm: This feels a little better even now.

Top of the head: What if it is enough I am heading in the right direction?

Take a breath.

Rate how strong the feeling is now from 0 (not strong at all) to 10 (extremely strong).

If this Bridging Round does not feel true for you, then go back and redo the first round a few more times. At some point, you can do this round, and it will feel truer for you. That is what you are looking for. When it feels truer, it is a great indicator you are moving in the right direction.

I recommend this three-part tapping sequence in this order to maximize the potential transformation of Rant Tapping.

Now let's jump to some very direct Rant Tapping sequences. If you begin this sequence and you notice guilt is still surfacing, go back and utilize tapping sequence #1 (Attending to Guilt about Rant Tapping) before these next sequences. We will turn the dial up on this next tapping sequence, so get ready for that. Just keep tapping through these sequences until you feel soothed.

Let's talk about gaslighting first.

According to Dr. George Simon, Ph.D., of the Counseling Resource in his article, "*Gaslighting as a Manipulation Tactic: What It Is, Who Does It, And Why?*" [6]

"Gaslighting is a sophisticated manipulation tactic which certain types of personalities use to create doubt in the minds of others. Here is how it works and what to watch out for:

"In a stage play and suspense thriller from the 1930s entitled Gas Light, a conniving husband tries to make the wife he wishes to get rid of think she is losing her mind by making subtle changes in her environment, including slowly and steadily dimming the flame on a gas lamp.

In recent years, the term 'gaslighting' has come to be applied to attempts by certain kinds of personalities, especially psychopaths—who are among the personalities most adept at sophisticated tactics of manipulation—to create so much doubt in the minds of their targets of exploitation that the victim no longer trusts their own judgment about things and buys into the assertions of the manipulator, thus coming under their power and control."

If you suspect you are being gaslighted, please seek professional help from a trained psychotherapist.

Tapping Sequence #4: Rant Tapping for Gaslighting

I have found Rant Tapping to be effective with clients to release a lot of their confusion that can turn to rage when dealing with someone who has been gaslighting them. Many people use gaslighting without being conscious they are doing it. You don't have to be dealing with a psychopath to be gaslighted. Use this sequence if you notice you doubt yourself with someone a lot and mistrust your own truth.

Think about someone you feel has wronged you. Someone who never apologized for things they did and turn it around to blame you. You start off the conversation knowing you have a point, and by the end of the conversation, your head is spinning. Confused and uncertain, you believe, on some level, it is your fault. You just know something's not right here, but you cannot quite put your finger on it.

What feeling is attached to this?

Rate how strong the feeling is from 0 (not strong at all) to 10 (extremely strong).

Now use the following script and edit it as you need to. If something pops up in your head that feels more accurate than what the script says, then say what is truer for you instead. This will help you target what is happening to you. Your brain will let you know when and where to change words for accuracy.

We go right to the eyebrow with Rant Tapping and start with the unedited truth.

Eyebrow: Oh, my God.

Side of the eye: What just happened?

Under the eye: What the hell?

Under the nose: Are you kidding me?

Chin point: I feel like I am crazy.

Collarbone: I started thinking I had a point.

Under the arm: How is it, I am wrong again?

Top of the head: They never take ownership.

Eyebrow: It is never their fucking fault.

Side of the eye: This is insane.

Under the eye: I am so tired of feeling this way.

Under the nose: Here I am again.

Chin point: Confused. Upset. Pissed.

Collarbone: And now I am feeling bad about me.

Under the arm: How is it possible they are never wrong?

Top of the head: How can they be that unreasonable?

Eyebrow: What the fuck!

185

Side of the eye: This is such bullshit.

Under the eye: This is crazy making.

Under the nose: What a nightmare.

Chin point: This is crazy.

Collarbone: I feel like I am losing it.

Under the arm: I feel like I am nuts, but I know I am not.

Top of the head: I am so tired of this.

Eyebrow: They always have an answer.

Side of the eye: And that answer is that it is always my fault.

Under the eye: What the fuck!

Under the nose: This is total bullshit.

Chin point: What a fucking jerk.

Collarbone: I will never win with this.

Under the arm: They will never hear me.

Top of the head: No wonder I feel crazy.

Eyebrow: No wonder I doubt myself.

Side of the eye: I am trying to get apple juice from an orange tree.

Under the eye: I will never win these battles.

Under the nose: They cannot hear me.

Chin point: They are not capable of it.

Collarbone: I am wasting my breath with them.

Under the arm: I am trying to be heard by someone who cannot hear me.

186

Top of the head: I have seen this pattern before.

Eyebrow: It is such crazy making.

Side of the eye: I learned this bullshit a long time ago.

Under the eye: I try to get people to hear me that can never hear me.

Under the nose: They are nuts.

Chin point: I am nuts for trying to get them to hear me.

Collarbone: I am so pissed.

Under the arm: I am so tired of this bullshit.

Top of the head: These arguments are exhausting.

Eyebrow: They are depleting.

Side of the Eye: I am so tired of feeling emotionally bullied.

Under the eye: I want to stop this, but I am not sure how.

Under the nose: So, what can I do?

Chin point: I cannot believe they never see my side of things.

Collarbone: Maybe they are fucking incapable of it, but it still pisses me off.

Under the arm: Like a moth to the flame, I go where I will lose again and again.

Top of the head: In more reflective moments, I know it is better to stop my part in this craziness.

Eyebrow: I just get sucked back in.

Side of the eye: This is such bullshit.

Under the eye: I cannot believe I am back here again.

187

Under the Nose: What if I can stop judging myself for this?

Chin point: What if this is the best place to start?

Collarbone: I am caught up in a dysfunctional pattern with them.

Under the arm: I actually own my anger right now.

Top of the head: I am allowing myself to feel this.

Eyebrow: I have been stuffing my anger for way too long.

Side of the eye: What if by owning this and finally allowing myself my feelings...

Under the eye: I can actually get to the other side of them?

Under the Nose: What if I can take ownership of myself?

Chin point: I need not apologize to them.

Collarbone: It might help to consider apologizing to myself.

Under the arm: What if by owning my part to myself only...

Top of the head: I can actually create some inner change for me?

Take a breath.

Rate how strong the feeling is now from 0 (not strong at all) to 10 (extremely strong).

If the feeling is stronger, it means you have targeted the emotions. Go back and do the tapping sequence as often as you need to until you feel soothed.

Notice which statement in this script feels more true or less true. If the statements expressing more anger feel true, keep tapping until they either feel less true when you rate them, or they have little emotional charge to them. This is a great indicator you are moving in the right direction and releasing suppressed emotions.

Once you feel soothed and your number is two or below, go to the next round.
Now let's round this out with a Bridging Round.

Tapping Sequence #5: Bridging Round to the Positive

Eyebrow: What if the best thing I can do is consider forgiving myself?
Side of the eye: What if I do have a right to my feelings, no matter what they taught me?
Under the eye: What if I can let myself have my own feelings?
Under the nose: I am hurt and confused, but it is not working on getting them to hear me.
Chin point: What if I really need to hear myself?
Collarbone: What if this is the place to start?
Under the arm: I may not understand how to do this yet...
Top of the head: What if I am starting to right now?

Eyebrow: I want to hear myself.
Side of the eye: But this sure feels foreign.
Under the eye: I have spent most of my life paying attention to everyone's feelings but
mine.
Under the Nose: What if I can learn to stay present with myself and my feelings?
Chin point: What if by doing this, I honor myself?

189

Collarbone: What if by learning to honor me...
Under the arm: I end up no longer needing anyone else to do it for me?
Top of the head: I would like to feel more empowered.

Eyebrow: I am not sure how to do this yet, but what if this is a start?
Side of the eye: This is a different way of seeing things.
Under the eye: I learned to treat myself the way they treated me.
Under the nose: So, what if this person is mirroring this to me?
Chin point: I need not like them.
Collarbone: I need not like what they have done.
Under the arm: Not at all.
Top of the head: But what if I can be even a little open to what I can learn here?

Eyebrow: What if I am getting a picture of how I have been treating myself?
Side of the eye: What if no matter how crazy this person is, it is a mirror of how I treat myself inside?
Under the eye: It may be too soon to believe this, but what if this might be true?
Under the Nose: What if I need not blame myself for this?
Chin point: I have done that enough to last me a lifetime.
Collarbone: What if I see this is the path to freedom?
Under the arm: I cannot change them. That is clear.
Top of the head: What if it starts with me? When I am ready.

Eyebrow: What if right now I can honor all of my feelings?
Side of the eye: What if I can see this as a gift I can give myself?
Under the eye: What if this is the path to true freedom?
Under the Nose: What if I can get there over time?

190

Chin point: What if it all starts with me considering allowing myself ALL of my feelings?
Collarbone: No matter what they are.
Under the arm: I need not believe this yet.
Top of the head: What if I can be open to this idea for now?
Eyebrow: What if by creating a tiny opening here in my beliefs, that is enough?
Side of the eye: It starts with me listening.
Under the eye: I do not listen to myself.
Under the nose: I was not listened too.
Chin point: What if, like anything new, I can learn how to listen?
Collarbone: I like this idea, whether I believe it yet or not.
Under the arm: I like that I can learn to empower myself.
Top of the head: I like that I can learn this.

Eyebrow: I enjoy knowing this might be possible.
Side of the eye: It might take me a while.
Under the eye: I have to unlearn things.
Under the Nose: What if I can get some traction with this?
Chin point: What if I am not alone?
Collarbone: What if there is help for me?
Under the arm: What if I can learn this over time?
Top of the head: I need not have this all figured out today.

Eyebrow: I like this idea, even if I do not believe it yet.
Side of the eye: What if there's some truth in this?
Under the eye: What if I can consider this and see what comes?
Under the nose: And what if the outcome of shifting myself is that I see positive shifts?
Chin point: I like this idea a lot.
Collarbone: I enjoy putting less pressure on myself.
Under the arm: This feels a little better even now.
Top of the head: What if it is enough I am heading in the right direction, even if just a little right now?

191

Take a breath.
Rate how strong the feeling is now from 0 (not strong at all) to 10 (extremely strong).

If the feeling is stronger, it means you have targeted the emotions. Go back and do the tapping sequence as often as you need to until you feel soothed, and these bridging statements feel true for you. This is a great indicator you are moving in the right direction, and you are shifting your negative beliefs around this.

Rant tapping can go so much deeper than this, especially when working with a professional. I consider Rant Tapping a lifesaver. This technique alone has the power to shift consciousness and release stuck emotions that create a buildup of energy in their energy systems.

I have used Rant Tapping when I have been hiking, which helps to move the energy through the body while moving and tapping. I have found it to be transformational.

Think of it this way. When you allow yourself to access your emotions—safely and healthfully—you become more emotionally fit and thus more emotionally intelligent. You learn to make better choices in your life. You can better decide where you want to spend your precious energy.

By pausing more often before getting caught up in reaction, you can decide if you want to engage or not. You become responsible for yourself, and you no longer feel so victimized by others. You're better able to practice Eckhart Tolle's idea of "watching the thinker." You become detached in the most empowering way.

I highly recommend you seek someone who can help you with these tapping techniques if you want emotional liberation, intelligence, and fitness, it will be worth it.

Now let's move on to another one of my favorite techniques, Argue Tapping. A highly effective way to learn to use your negative thoughts to free yourself emotionally. You can learn to release the limiting beliefs that keep you from moving forward, so it feels good to you.

Chapter Summary

Rant tapping is the most effective technique I know of that allows you to free yourself from what can feel like the darkest of emotions, rage, hatred, terror, etc.

It provides a safe way to move through any emotion you feel, which allows you to free yourself from feeling bad about these emotions.

You realize it is part of being human, feeling. Over time, more uplifting and supporting thoughts replace negative thought patterns.

This shows that your physiology is changing, which allows for lasting change to take place. Life becomes more hopeful and even positive and uplifting, all the while knowing that what feels like negative emotion will not last.

It will pass through, and you'll feel more at ease.

Argue Tapping

What Is Argue Tapping?

We each have different battles that go on inside of us. They described this inner battle during Deepak Chopra and Oprah Winfrey's meditation series, *Hope in Uncertain Times.* Oprah quotes American inspirational speaker and author, Iyanla Vanzant. from an interview she conducted with Vanzant on Super Soul Sunday:

> "There's no greater battle in life than the battle between the parts of you that want to be healed and the parts of you that are comfortable, and content being broken.

> "We all have an inner battle between these parts with their conflicting desires."

Argue Tapping neutralizes these inner battles and conflicts.

With this technique, you bring your inner argument into your conscious awareness. As you do this, you tap back and forth between the two parts of yourself that are in conflict. Argue Tapping lightens and releases your conflicts.

I always tell my clients it is the tennis match that goes on inside of your head.

When Is It Effective to Use Argue Tapping?

Argue Tapping is my favorite technique when I notice a client has an internal conflict. I can hear the back and forth battle they are having within themselves.

A superb example of this shows up in close personal relationships. I have experienced this myself, and I have had many clients who battle within about whether to stay in a relationship when they feel their needs are not getting met. They want more connection, and they are not getting it. So, the battle becomes, do I stay, or do I go?

It is a major conflict, so we tap on the conflict. Here is how it would sound.

Argue Tapping on Relationship Conflict: To Stay or Go

Karate Chop: Even though I want to leave because I have had it, but I cannot go, I acknowledge I feel this way.

Karate Chop: Even though I want to leave, and I need to leave, but I cannot leave, I see I have a major conflict here. I accept myself and my feelings now.

Karate Chop: Even though I want to leave, and I cannot leave, I accept myself anyway.

Eyebrow: I need to leave.

Side of the Eye: I cannot leave.

Under the Eye: I really need to leave.

Under the Nose: I cannot leave.

Chin Point: I really need to leave. I am sick of this.

Collarbone: So why do I keep staying?

Under the Arm: I need to leave.

Top of the Head: I cannot leave.

Eyebrow: I need to go.

Side of the Eye: I cannot go.

Under the Eye: I am tired of this.

Under the Nose: I am not tired enough.

Chin Point: I need to leave.

Collarbone: I cannot leave.

Under the Arm: I will leave.

Top of the Head: No, I won't.

In this quick tapping example, if you say it out loud and tap while you do it, you will hear the inner conflict. When you have your own inner conflict going on, this technique brings it out into the open. When you hear yourself say it out loud, it loses its grip on you. I tell my clients to Argue Tap until they laugh about it.

What Are the Benefits of Argue Tapping?

You can have the most serious inner battle going on, and if you keep tapping on it, eventually you will laugh about it. It feels ridiculous to you in the best way. Once you either laugh or saying to yourself some variation of, "This is silly," you have created what we call in the Tapping world a cognitive shift.

EFT Founder Gary Craig defines a cognitive shift from his article, "*Cognitive Shifts - Belief Changes Within EFT - New Insights, Behaviors & Beliefs Are Routine With EFT.* "

"When a client has a new insight, exhibits new behavior, or demonstrates a new belief about their issue, then something significant has shifted in their perception and this is seen as evidence that emotional healing or growth has occurred."[7]

Argue Tapping is a powerful technique with the ability to create a cognitive shift because you are bringing an inner argument to the surface and out in the open. When you speak both sides of the argument out loud, you can better hear and feel how this internal arguing creates stress in your life.

By learning of the inner argument while using Argue Tapping, you benefit by releasing the stress around the inner conflict more quickly. The quicker you can release the stress, the quicker you will free up your creative mind to come up with a solution.

Let's go back to the example of not feeling you're getting your needs met in a relationship. Once you clear your central argument about whether to stay or to go. You will find you can see the relationship in a different light. You realize that not getting your needs met is really a mirror into your early wounding as a child. As you tap to release the belief that your needs don't get met, you create the space for you to meet your own needs. The amazing part is now that you no longer grasp for your partner to meet your needs, they might start to give "magically" more to you because energetically you are free from the burden of your past.

Here are examples of how to best use the Argue Tapping technique:

Exercise #1 You Cannot Make a Decision About Something

1) Call to mind something you are unable to decide about.
2) Now say out loud, "I can't decide about this."
3) Rate how true this feels on the 0–10 Scale (0 = Not true; and 10 = Totally true).
4) Now try the following tapping script.

Karate Chop:

Even though I am so confused about this and I cannot decide what to do here, I choose to

acknowledge I feel this way.

Karate Chop:

Even though I am confused, and I mean I am really confused about this, I want to accept me anyway.

Karate Chop:

Even though I am really confused, and I just cannot seem to decide here, I am open to not

feeling confused.

Eyebrow: I am really confused.

Side of the Eye: I cannot decide.

Under the Eye: I can decide

Under the Nose: No, I cannot.

Chin Point: I would have by now.

Collarbone: I can get to a decision.

Under the Arm: No, I cannot.

Top of the Head: Yes, I can.

Eyebrow: No, I cannot.

Side of the Eye: I am too confused.

Under the Eye: I cannot decide.

Under the Nose: What if I can?

Chin Point: No, I cannot.

Collarbone: What if I can?

199

Under the Arm: No, I cannot.

Top of the Head: What if I can decide once I release the stress?

Eyebrow: That will not work.

Side of the Eye: What if it can?

Under the Eye: I cannot decide.

Under the Nose: What if the stress is in the way of me deciding?

Chin Point: What???

Collarbone: What does that even mean?

Under the Arm: What if the pressure I am putting on myself to decide is the very thing in my way?

Top of the Head: Now, that is an interesting concept.

Eyebrow: But I still cannot decide.

Side of the Eye: What if I can get clearer once I release all this pressure I feel about having to decide?

Under the Eye: That will not make a difference.

Under the Nose: What if it can make all the difference?

Chin Point: No, it cannot.

Collarbone: What if it can?

Under the Arm: I need to decide.

Top of the Head: But I cannot right now.

Eyebrow: I need to decide.

Side of the Eye: I cannot.

Under the Eye: Yes, I can.

Under the Nose: No, I cannot.

Chin Point: Yes, I can.

Collarbone: No, I cannot.

Under the Arm: Yes, I can.

Top of the Head: No, I cannot.

Eyebrow: What if the first thing I need to do here is to release the pressure and the stress?

Side of the Eye: What if by releasing the pressure and the stress, a great decision can come?

Under the Eye: What if this is true?

Under the Nose: I have been putting this pressure on myself to decide and I cannot.

Chin Point: So, what if I consider that by releasing the judgment and pressure...

Collarbone: A brilliant decision might come with ease?

Under the Arm: That will not happen.

Top of the Head: What if it can?

Eyebrow: Maybe it can.

Side of the Eye: What if I can consider this might be possible?

Under the Eye: That idea feels better.

Under the Nose: What if it is possible?

Chin Point: I like that it is possible.

Collarbone: What if the belief I can't decide is causing me so much pressure?

Under the Arm: Let me try this.

Top of the Head: And see what happens.

201

Eyebrow: I cannot decide.

Side of the Eye: I can decide.

Under the Eye: I cannot decide.

Under the Nose: I can decide.

Chin Point: I cannot decide yet.

Collarbone: But I will be able to decide.

Under the Arm: I cannot decide yet.

Top of the Head: But I will be able to decide.

Eyebrow: I cannot decide.

Side of the Eye: Yes, I can.

Under the Eye: I cannot decide.

Under the Nose: Yes, I can.

Chin Point: I cannot decide.

Collarbone: Yes, I can.

Under the Arm: I cannot decide.

Top of the Head: Oh yes, I can.

Eyebrow: What if by softening this pressure to decide...

Side of the Eye: An inspired thought comes that helps me to decide?

Under the Eye: What if as I release some of this pressure...

Under the Nose: I open myself up to this possibility?

Chin Point: What if I made decisions through me rather than by me?

Collarbone: What if this really could be possible?

Under the Arm: What if I need not figure this out?

Top of the Head: What if the answer I need comes with ease, as I feel relieved of this pressure?

Re-rate the statement "I cannot decide about this" using that scale of 0–10.

Notice if your number has dropped. If, when you first said, *"I cannot decide about this,"* you rated it as a nine because it felt true, and now it feels less true, so say you are at a 5, then you are moving in the right direction. Keep tapping on this sequence until your number is between a 0–3.

If the numbers don't work for you, notice if you feel lighter when you say the statement, "I can't decide about this." Does this statement feel lighter in your body (which means it feels less true,) or does it feel heavier (meaning it feels more true)?

Again, I recommend you Argue Tap on this until it feels ridiculous to you.

Exercise #2 Love/Hate Situations

1) Call to mind someone or some situation you feel intense conflict about. For this exercise, I will use a person.
2) Now say out loud, "I love them, and I hate them."
3) Rate how true this feels on the 0–10 Scale (0 = Not true; 10 = Totally true).
4) Now follow the tapping script below.

Karate Chop:

Even though I feel so conflicted, and I love them, and I hate them, I acknowledge I feel this way.

203

Karate Chop:

Even though I love them, and I hate them, but I am not supposed to hate anyone, I accept that I have this conflict.

Karate Chop:

Even though I love them, and I hate them, and I feel guilty saying I hate them because I am supposed to love them, I acknowledge my conflicted feelings.

Eyebrow: I love them.

Side of the Eye: No, I hate them.

Under the Eye: I love them.

Under the Nose: No, I hate them.

Chin Point: I love them.

Collarbone: No, I hate them.

Under the Arm: I love them.

Top of the Head: I hate them.

Eyebrow: I love them.

Side of the Eye: But I hate them right now.

Under the Eye: I love them.

Under the Nose: And I hate them right now.

Chin Point: I love them.

Collarbone: And I hate them right now.

Under the Arm: I love them.

Top of the Head: I hate them, too.

Eyebrow: Both are true.

Side of the Eye: I love them.

Under the Eye: Right now, I just hate them.

Under the Nose: I love them.

Chin Point: I hate them right now.

Collarbone: I love them.

Under the Arm: And I hate them right now.

Top of the Head: I love them.

Eyebrow: And I hate their behavior.

Side of the Eye: I love them.

Under the Eye: I hate what they did.

Under the Nose: I love them.

Chin Point: I hate what they did.

Collarbone: I love them.

Under the Arm: I hate what they did.

Top of the Head: I love them.

Eyebrow: I hate what they did.

Side of the Eye: What if I can open to healing this now?

Under the Eye: I do not want to feel hatred, but I do right now.

Under the Nose: What if, as shocking as this may sound...

Chin Point: There's nothing wrong with feeling hatred right now?

Collarbone: I know I do not want to stay stuck in this long term.

Under the Arm: What if there's nothing wrong with feeling hatred?

205

Top of the Head: What if it is an indicator of how disempowered I feel?

Eyebrow: Good people feel hatred sometimes.

Side of the Eye: It is letting me know I feel disempowered.

Under the Eye: What if by acknowledging my hatred, I release it?

Under the Nose: I need not hurt anyone by doing this, including myself.

Chin Point: Sometimes, I feel hatred.

Collarbone: This does not mean I have to act on it.

Under the Arm: What if by acknowledging the hatred, and tapping through it, it helps me to release it?

Top of the Head: It is not the hatred itself that is the problem.

Eyebrow: I need not act on it.

Side of the Eye: I can just feel it and tap through it, so I can complete this feeling.

Under the Eye: What if by completing this feeling in this safe way, where no one gets hurt, I begin not to feel it anymore?

Under the Nose: What if judging myself for feeling hatred is the very thing that holds it in place?

Chin Point: I am not bad for feeling hatred.

Collarbone: It is just where I am at right now.

Under the Arm: The truth is I am hurt, and I believe I am disempowered here.

Top of the Head: What if I am not disempowered?

206

Eyebrow: What if by empowering myself to feel fully...

Side of the Eye: I am doing the best thing I can for myself?

Under the Eye: I am completing a feeling.

Under the Nose: What if by completing a feeling, I release it, so it no longer has power over me?

Chin Point: I like this idea a lot.

Collarbone: I need not stay stuck here.

Under the Arm: I can complete my feelings no matter what they are.

Top of the Head: And by doing this, I set myself and this person free.

Eyebrow: I like this idea a lot.

Side of the Eye: I am just feeling and releasing.

Under the Eye: This is better for me.

Under the Nose: Better for this person too.

Chin Point: Because it sets me free.

Collarbone: And then I am more empowered to deal with them more effectively.

Under the Arm: I like this idea a lot.

Top of the Head: Sometimes, I both love them and hate them, and that is okay.

Eyebrow: I will not stay stuck in the hatred when I fully feel it.

Side of the Eye: This feels liberating.

Under the Eye: This feels more freeing.

207

Under the Nose: I am freer to feel fully.

Chin Point: Without all the judgment.

Collarbone: I am healing myself by feeling fully.

Under the Arm: I like this idea a lot.

Top of the Head: And I am healing myself right now.

Re-rate the statement "I love them, and I hate them" using the same scale of 0–10.

Notice if your number has dropped. If, when you first said, *"I love them, and I hate them,"* you rated it as a nine because it felt true, and now it feels less true, so say you are at a 5, then you are moving the right direction. Keep tapping on this sequence until your number is between a 0–3.

If the numbers don't work for you, just notice if you feel lighter when you say the statement, "I love them and hate them." Does this statement feel lighter (this means it feels less true), or heavier (this means it feels more true)?

Again, I recommend you Argue Tap on this until it feels ridiculous to you.

Exercise #3 Money – There's Not Enough

There are many benefits to Argue Tapping on your financial situation and money. If your financial situation feels less abundant than you would like, you may have stuck energy or limiting beliefs regarding money you would benefit from clearing out.

We often blame ourselves for our lack of money. Telling ourselves we do not have what it takes or are missing the money gene. We fall back on limiting beliefs we learned early in life around money.

These beliefs can keep us from allowing more into our lives in the form of money when this gets released, you are more open to allowing more to flow into your experience.

Note sometimes, what we want, does not come into our experience no matter how often we have tapped or released limiting beliefs. When this happens, consider:

What if money isn't coming into your experience in the way you think it should, because you are being guided and directed to something even greater? What if you are being directed to release the programming, you learned from the people and society you are immersed in, on how money should be or look? What if you are being opened up to a greater experience around money different from how society tells you money should show up for you?

Even if your financial situation feels abundant, you may experience Forbidden Emotions about money, and the desire to bring more into your life. Maybe you feel greedy or guilty for wanting more when you already have more than most, for example.

1) Call to mind your financial life. Let's say it is not where you want it to be. You want to make more money and bring more money into your experience, and despite your best efforts, it is not happening for you.

2) Now say out loud, "I want more money in my life."

3) Now I want you to say it again and notice what pops into your head after you say it. Your tail-enders or your current truths. An example is: *"I want more money in my life,"* and the little voice in your head says, *"Yeah, but I'll never have enough."* This is your tail-ender...your current true affirmation. *"I'll never have enough."*

4) Rate how true your tail-ender statement "I will never have enough" feels on the 0–10 Scale (0 = Not true; 10 = Totally true).

209

5) Now try the following tapping script.

Karate Chop:

Even though deep down, I do not believe I will ever have enough, I acknowledge this is my current truth.

Karate Chop:

Even though this feels true for me, that I will never have enough, and even though I dislike it, I acknowledge I have this conflict.

Karate Chop:

Even though I do not believe I will ever have enough, I want to accept myself anyway.

.

Eyebrow: I want more money.

Side of the Eye: This really is true.

Under the Eye: But deep down, I do not believe I ever will have enough.

Under the Nose: Never mind more than enough.

Chin Point: I will never have enough.

Collarbone: What if I can?

Under the Arm: That is a joke. I will never have enough.

Top of the Head: I want more money in my life.

Eyebrow: I may want more, but I will never have more.

Side of the Eye: This is so frustrating.

Under the Eye: I really, really want more money in my life.

Under the Nose: But I do not really believe I will ever have more.

Chin Point: That is scary because if I do not believe I will have more, I never will.

Collarbone: What if I can change this belief?

Under the Arm: I have tried so often already.

Top of the Head: And yet here I am, still not having enough.

Eyebrow: I want more money in my life.

Side of the Eye: What is wrong with me I can't create more?

Under the Eye: I want more money, and I cannot create it.

Under the Nose: I hear a major conflict here.

Chin Point: I want more money in my life.

Collarbone: I will never have more.

Under the Arm: I want more.

Top of the Head: Yeah, but I never get more.

Eyebrow: What if I can get more?

Side of the Eye: I don't believe it. It would have happened by now.

Under the Eye: I want more, and I cannot get it.

Under the Nose: I want more.

Chin Point: I will never get it.

Collarbone: I want more, and yet I am convinced I will never get it.

Under the Arm: I have these two conflicting thoughts.

211

Top of the Head: I know I really, really, really want more.

Eyebrow: Yet my truer belief is that I will never have more.

Side of the Eye: I want more.

Under the Eye: I will never have more.

Under the Nose: I want more.

Chin Point: I will never have more.

Collarbone: I want more.

Under the Arm: I will never have more.

Top of the Head: I want more.

Eyebrow: I will never have more.

Side of the Eye: I want more.

Under the Eye: I will never have more.

Under the Nose: I want more.

Chin Point: I will never have more.

Collarbone: I want more.

Under the Arm: I will never have more.

Top of the Head: But what if I can change my belief so I believe I can have more?

Eyebrow: Can I have it then?

Side of the Eye: I want more.

Under the Eye: And what if I can have more?

Under the Nose: What if I can change the belief I will never have more?

Chin Point: It really is just a belief.

Collarbone: What if I can really change it?

Under the Arm: What if I am changing this belief right now?

Top of the Head: What if, over time, I can soften the belief I will never have more?

Eyebrow: And strengthen the belief I can have more?

Side of the Eye: What if that is possible?

Under the Eye: What if I can get there?

Under the Nose: I like this idea a lot.

Chin Point: I will never have more.

Collarbone: What if I can?

Under the Arm: I will never have more.

Top of the Head: What if I can?

Eyebrow: I will never have more.

Side of the Eye: What if I can?

Under the Eye: I will never have more.

Under the Nose: Yes, I can.

Chin Point: No, I cannot.

Collarbone: Yes, I can.

Under the Arm: No, I cannot.

Top of the Head: Yes, I can.

Eyebrow: I like the idea that I can have more.

Side of the Eye: I like the idea that I can change my belief about this.

213

Under the Eye: I like the idea that by changing my belief, I can change my reality.

Under the Nose: I like this idea a lot.

Chin Point: In fact, I love this idea.

Collarbone: What if it is true?

Under the Arm: That I can change the belief I will never have more...

Top of the Head: Over to believing I can have more?

Eyebrow: What if it is already feeling even a bit more possible?

Side of the Eye: What if this is the best thing I can do?

Under the Eye: I need not try harder or do more.

Under the Nose: I need to work on shifting my beliefs that do not serve me.

Chin Point: To beliefs that do serve me.

Collarbone: What if I can shift my beliefs more and more?

Under the Arm: What if I really can have more?

Top of the Head: What if this feels a little more possible even now?

Eyebrow: What if I am on my way to having more?

Side of the Eye: I like this thought a lot.

Under the Eye: This thought feels better.

Under the Nose: What if I can believe this thought more and more?

Chin Point: What if I notice I am feeling more hopeful?

Collarbone: What if this is moving me in the right direction?

Under the Arm: What if I am already feeling a little better and lighter right now?

Top of the Head: What if this is what I need to do?

Eyebrow: What if by softening the belief I will never have more...

Side of the Eye: I loosen this belief's grip on me?

Under the Eye: And what if by doing this, I notice I feel better?

Under the Nose: What if feeling better draws better things into my life?

Chin Point: What if I am on my way?

Collarbone: What if this Argue Tapping is working?

Under the Arm: What if I can do this any time I feel resistance?

Top of the Head: And the more I interrupt the belief I cannot have more...

Eyebrow: The more the belief and reality of having more flows into my life?

Side of the Eye: It cannot hurt to believe this is possible.

Under the Eye: What if it helps?

Under the Nose: What if I am getting closer?

Chin Point: What if I felt lighter right now?

Collarbone: What if I am on my way?

Under the Arm: I like this idea a lot.

Top of the Head: This idea sure feels better.

215

Eyebrow: Let me try this again.

Side of the Eye: I will never have more.

Under the Eye: I can have more.

Under the Nose: I will never have more.

Chin Point: I will have more.

Collarbone: I will never have more.

Under the Arm: I can have more.

Top of the Head: I will never have more.

Eyebrow: I will have more.

Side of the Eye: I cannot have more.

Under the Eye: I can have more.

Under the Nose: I cannot have more.

Chin Point: I will have more.

Collarbone: I cannot have more.

Under the Arm: I can have more.

Top of the Head: And I am on my way to more right now.

Eyebrow: I love knowing I can shift my beliefs.

Side of the Eye: I understand I might not see outward shifts immediately.

Under the Eye: But I love that as I am shifting my inner beliefs...

Under the Nose: My outer world will eventually follow.

Chin Point: I like this idea a lot.

Collarbone: I can have more.

Under the Arm: I can get to where I really believe this.

Top of the Head: And I stepped on that path just now.

Eyebrow: What if after all of this, I realize that I've been grasping for more...

Side of the Eye: And what does more really mean anyway?

Under the Eye: What if there is another way to see having more?

Under the Nose: What if I feel content as things are right now?

Chin Point: What if I feel more peace about money?

Collarbone: What if by feeling more peace, I feel a lot freer? What if I see money in a fresh way?

Under the Arm: A way that brings me more peace?

Top of the Head: What if this really works for me?

Re-rate the statement "I will never have enough" using the same scale of 0–10.

Notice if your number has dropped. If, when you first said, *"I will never have more,"* you rated it a nine because it felt true, and now it feels less true, so you rate it at a 5, then you are moving in the right direction. Keep tapping on this sequence until your number is between a 0–3.

If the numbers don't work for you, notice if you feel lighter when you say the statement, "I'll never have more." Does this statement feel lighter after tapping (this suggests it feels less true) or heavier (this suggests it feels more true)?

Again, I recommend you Argue Tap on this until it feels ridiculous to you.

When you Argue Tap, you are training your brain to follow a negative thought with a positive thought. The more you Argue Tap on any conflict, the more you will notice, as your original limiting thought comes to mind, your brain firing off positive follow-up thoughts.

This creates a cognitive shift. Your mind will choose the positive more often. When this happens, you will eventually notice what shows up in your outside world reflects your newly established positive inner experience. What you thought you wanted is replaced with something even better than you could imagine.

Pick any topic you have a conflict in, try Argue Tapping on it, and see what changes for you.

Chapter Summary

Argue Tapping, like Rant Tapping, is tapping used under specific circumstances when any issue or person poses a conflict for you.

When the brain remains in conflict over something, the conflicting thoughts play off of each other and neutralize each other. When this continues, you can find yourself stuck in a negative pattern of behavior without moving through it. Argue Tapping does two important things, it trains the brain to follow a negative thought with a positive one. It interrupts the negative thought pattern.

You may want something to change, which is true, but when you have a limiting belief, it can't change, this is the perfect time to use Argue Tapping.

When you say out loud the two competing thoughts, while tapping, you're more likely to notice how the negative thoughts surrounding an issue or persons shift and feel lighter and thus less true.

By continuing to use this technique until you notice the negative thought feels less and less true, you've effectively broken up this conflict. You can take steps forward without the conflict taking over.

Lifelong Process

"There's nothing like returning to a place that remains unchanged to find all the ways in which you yourself have altered." ~ Nelson Mandela

I spent decades with the belief that if I just worked hard enough, if I just figured out what was in my way, if I just... if I just... if I just... then I would arrive. I would be complete.

You have likely heard quotes about enjoying the journey, but do you believe this? Do you believe that life is a journey you will never get done, never finish, never complete?

Depending on your religious affiliation, or your spiritual beliefs, you really will never do it, even in death. If you believe you go on after death, then you are never completed. If you believe there's nothing after death, then I invite you to consider that you have this one life to live and you will not get it all done in this lifetime. You will always have an inner longing for desires to come into being, so it's still a journey, but will you ever "arrive"?

I saw an interview with Clint Eastwood, who at the time was eighty-four. They asked if he would ever retire and I remember the look on his face. He looked perplexed, as if it had never occurred to him to retire. He went on to ask, "Why would I do that? I love what I'm doing."

He said that there's always something new he wants to do or try, so he will never be done. This speaks to tapping. This is a tool you will have with you for the rest of your life to help you through the bumps and turns that life can take.

Sometimes it seems like we have gone off track, but have we really? Life will always present challenges that seem like we have gone off track, but if we're open to it, maybe we need to learn something. Tapping can help you to navigate through any challenges in life with more grace and ease.

Embracing this as a lifelong process you need not get done or get right helps in the progress you can make with tapping. Let me add, this is a great thing to tap on. The releasing of the need to do it and get it right is a tappable issue. You may need to tap on this a few times.

Let's do a tapping exercise on this right now!

Tapping Exercise: You Do not Need to Get It Done or Get It Right

Please take responsibility for yourself and keep tapping if strong emotion surfaces until you feel soothed.

Karate Chop:
Even though I have this belief to get this right and that I have to do this, I learned this a long time ago, I choose to acknowledge I feel this way.

Karate Chop:
Even though I have this belief to get this right and I have to rid myself of all of my dysfunction, I want to accept myself anyway.

Karate Chop:
Even though I have this belief to be perfect, I have to get it right, I have to get this done, and I have to rid myself of all of my flaws, what if I can be open to accepting myself anyway?

Eyebrow: I have to get this right.

Side of the Eye: I have to.

221

Under the Eye: It is imperative I get this right.

Under the Nose: I am so messed up.

Chin Point: I am such a mess.

Collarbone: I have to get this right.

Under the Arm: I have to clean myself up.

Top of the Head: I am a mess, so this needs to be done.

Eyebrow: I learned this somewhere.

Side of the Eye: I have to get this right.

Under the Eye: I have to be perfect.

Under the Nose: Flaws are terrible.

Chin Point: They should be done away with.

Collarbone: They are not meant to be accepted.

Under the Arm: If you accept flaws, they will just get worse.

Top of the Head: Flaws are terrible.

Eyebrow: I have to get this right.

Side of the Eye: I have to do this.

Under the Eye: I have to be perfect.

Under the Nose: I believe this.

Chin Point: Man, it is a lot of pressure.

Collarbone: It is major pressure.

Under the Arm: I keep trying to be perfect.

Top of the Head: Trying to get this right.

Eyebrow: And here I am, still imperfect.

Side of the Eye: I am imperfect.

Under the Eye: Everyone else I know is perfect.

Under the Nose: The people that trained me to believe I need to be perfect are perfect.

Chin Point: Wait a minute. Are they?

Collarbone: Whose idea is it anyway that I need to be perfect?

Under the Arm: Is it a helpful belief?

Top of the Head: It sure feels like a ton of pressure.

Eyebrow: And pressure forms beautiful diamonds.

Side of the Eye: That is diamonds, that is not humans.

Under the Eye: Diamonds do not have feelings.

Under the Nose: Aren't I different?

Chin Point: Am I supposed to be perfect?

Collarbone: And by whose standard? Because there is not a worldwide standard.

Under the Arm: I am human, and we are not perfect.

Top of the Head: What if I can consider this idea?

Eyebrow: I am perfectly imperfect.

Side of the Eye: What if this is true?

Under the Eye: What if that is actually a good thing?

Under the Nose: What if my beauty is in my imperfections?

Chin Point: What if I am not meant to be perfect?

Collarbone: What if I am perfectly imperfect?

Under the Arm: I kind of like this idea.

223

Top of the Head: It feels like less pressure for sure.

Eyebrow: What if perfection is a myth?

Side of the Eye: What if I can learn to accept all of me?

Under the Eye: What if I can learn to appreciate and love my flaws?

Under the Nose: What if I am where I am supposed to be?

Chin Point: What if I will always be a work in progress?

Collarbone: What if I will never really get it done?

Under the Arm: What if that is why I am here?

Top of the Head: To learn and grow.

Eyebrow: I can learn from my mistakes if I choose to.

Side of the Eye: What if mistakes are good?

Under the Eye: They tell me I am in the game of life.

Under the Nose: I am not sitting on the sidelines.

Chin Point: What if growth and evolution is a lifelong process?

Collarbone: What if I will always evolve?

Under the Arm: What if I can embrace this idea?

Top of the Head: This idea may just feel better.

Eyebrow: I will always be a work in progress.

Side of the Eye: Perfection is really an illusion in the way they taught me.

Under the Eye: What if I will always be imperfect?

Under the Nose: What if I can make this okay?

Chin Point: I like this thought better.

Collarbone: It does feel lighter.

Under the Arm: I will always evolve.

Top of the Head: And this is a good thing.

Take a Breath.

Check in and see how you feel. For more relief, go back and tap on this sequence. Repeat this as often as needed. If you notice you feel lighter, that is a great indication you have changed your physiology and your momentum for the better. Results can vary among people, so just keep tapping.

Results Can Be Immediate but Not Always Dramatic

Years ago, clinical psychologist and founder and developer of the *Callahan Techniques® Thought Field Therapy, Roger J. Callahan, Ph.D.*, worked with a woman named Mary with a lifelong phobia of water. He tapped with her, and within a few minutes she had released her water phobia.

That was a dramatic result. I have had clients that have had dramatic results as referenced earlier in this book, but when I tapped, the results came over time and have always seemed more gradual. I still get results and continue to use tapping to keep myself "tuned up."

During my process, I "magically" seemed to stop doing habits of behavior not serving me. The first one I noticed was I had stopped making unreasonable comparisons of myself to others. If you remember, I used to compare myself and my life to movie stars and their lives. They seemed to have it all.

225

I remember one time my husband had said in my pre-tapping days when I was lamenting my plight in life, "Wow Marti, when you lose, you make sure you lose big." This was so true. I was comparing myself and my life to people in a profession I had no interest in being a part of. That is a surefire way to lose big because you start with an unreasonable comparison. Comparing is often something you can use to beat yourself up unconsciously.

When I caught myself comparing myself to others, I would use tapping to interrupt this pattern of comparing. I noticed the behavior had stopped. This was a shift and a big win for me. Often you notice these results first, meaning the behaviors you've minimized or stopped.

I also had this annoying 5–7-pound (2–3 kilos) weight fluctuation. This "magically" seemed to disappear. Although I never tapped on this directly, it was another great result.

One of my tapping mentors noticed her insomnia "magically" went away despite not even tapping on that issue for herself; she was just working with others. This speaks to Borrowing Benefits we can receive in tapping. Borrowing Benefits is where you tap along with someone else on their issues and you may benefit by clearing up something within yourself whether or not it is your direct issue.

These "wins" add up and your life changes for the better because you're building momentum by allowing more good feelings within you to come through. They now have the space to do so.

Overall, I notice how I continue to show up for myself by feeling and honoring my emotions more in areas where in the past I would have sabotaged myself. I notice my resistance of fear surfacing, and then I tap on it and this softens the fear which allows me to move forward because I'm shifting my physiology.

As you release more emotional blocks that carry a host of possible negative messaging with them, you will become more positive and optimistic without trying. It will become natural to look on the bright side more easily without the effort. You don't have to "try" to think positively or "try" to manifest good in your life. Pushing, effecting, and trying, becomes exhausting.

We all have a resting heart rate and I believe we also have a resting thought rate. When I first learned of my inner thoughts, it amazed me at how I felt like I had a cesspool of negative thinking going on inside of me. Once I tapped, I noticed and continue to notice that when I catch my resting thoughts, they are more positive than they used to be. If I notice my negative resting thoughts, I tap to attend to them and shift that. I will always be a work in progress. I invite you to realize this is true for you too. We're not really taught that we don't have to get it right and we'll never get it done.

When You Change What Happens Around You Changes

I want to address what can happen when you change. Like Nelson Mandela's quote, at the beginning of this chapter, you can notice you feel differently about people in your life. I have had many clients who go through a stage in their personal development where they notice that some of their relationships feel vastly different to them. It is as if someone has placed a microscope in front of their eyes and they notice how some of their relationships do not feel like they work for them anymore. They see the dysfunction in the relationships and they now want to distance themselves from these relationships. Sometimes clients get scared when this happens because they are afraid, they must rid themselves of these people, but this could not be further from the truth. It's also possible that they see these relationships as mirrors into themselves and where they need more tapping. These relationships can be the greatest teachers.

227

Whichever path you chose around relationships, as you release limiting beliefs, your self-esteem increases, and you value yourself more and want better for yourself. When you want better for yourself, you often first notice more things that do not work in your life anymore. You have new eyes. You see things anew. You have a fresh perspective, and you realize you have grown and changed.

The conditions you have been living in appear intolerable to you because you have become an alternative version of yourself. A light is shining on what no longer works in your life. The wonderful news is you have choices here. You can release the relationship, or you can see it as a roadmap on what to tap on. The feelings now surfacing are coming up so you can feel them through to their completion and release them.

When you release them, it changes you in a healthier way. People in your life have to change if you change because you are no longer an energetic match, so either they behave differently with you or they move along or you move along—and you will be okay with what happens.

Either way, you are a new version of yourself, and you will move on to your next up-leveling within yourself. If you keep up with tapping and use it when you need to, you will continue to evolve and change for the better. You can learn to embrace your own personal evolution that will continue throughout your life.

Be Patient

Impatience is resistance. Learning to be patient with yourself takes the pressure off having to get it right or be perfect. If you do not feel patient about this, it is a good thing to tap on. It is a tappable issue. Remember this, you will always be a work in progress, and you have a lot of company because we are all works in progress.

Below is another tapping sequence to use when you feel impatient with your progress.

Tapping Exercise: Releasing Impatience

Karate Chop:

Even though I am not changing fast enough, I choose to acknowledge I feel this way.

Karate Chop:

Even though I am seeing how far I have to go and not appreciating how far I have come, I choose to accept that I feel this way.

Karate Chop:

Even though I am impatient with my progress and I feel I should be farther along by now, I want to accept myself anyway now.

Eyebrow: Come on already.

Side of the Eye: How long is this going to take?

Under the Eye: I want to be over this already.

Under the Nose: I clear up something and something else surfaces.

Chin Point: What a pain in the ass.

Collarbone: I really hate this.

Under the Arm: I want to be further along already.

Top of the Head: My impatience is resistance.

Eyebrow: What?

Side of the Eye: Yes. My impatience is resistance.

Under the Eye: I have come a long way already.

Under the Nose: But I cannot see that when I am impatient.

229

Chin Point: I want things to shift more quickly.

Collarbone: It is not fast enough.

Under the Arm: What if I am missing a key here?

Top of the Head: What if I can move my focus to what has changed for me already?

Eyebrow: What if I feel better because I am seeing my progress?

Side of the Eye: What if by weighing in on my progress, I see more progress?

Under the Eye: What if the key is to see how far I have come already?

Under the Nose: What if I can appreciate that?

Chin Point: What if by appreciating what has shifted for me, I will feel better?

Collarbone: What if by feeling better, better things come?

Under the Arm: I learned a long time ago that the glass is half empty.

Top of the Head: This is how this shows up for me.

Eyebrow: More impatience.

Side of the Eye: More heaviness.

Under the Eye: It does not feel good to be impatient.

Under the Nose: That feels heavy.

Chin Point: I have felt heavy enough in my life.

Collarbone: I want to learn how to appreciate more.

Under the Arm: Why not?

Top of the Head: I have tried it the other way, and that feels bad.

Eyebrow: What if by learning to appreciate, more shows up to appreciate?

Side of the Eye: I like this idea a lot.

Under the Eye: What if the better I see it, the better it gets?

Under the Nose: What if I'm opening up to new possibilities as I practice focusing on what is shifting for me?

Chin Point: What if this is true?

Collarbone: I need not believe it yet.

Under the Arm: What if I can create an opening for this belief?

Top of the Head: Just a little crack in my limiting beliefs.

Eyebrow: What if this crack allows in a stream of possibilities?

Side of the Eye: What if I believe more and more that good is possible for me?

Under the Eye: What if I will notice more evidence of the changes within me?

Under the Nose: What if these internal changes reflect in my external life?

Chin Point: What if greater inspiration, guidance, and direction comes?

Collarbone: What if more possibilities come?

Under the Arm: What if I see more evidence that my life is improving?

231

Top of the Head: What if I will expect more wonderful things for me?

Eyebrow: What if I believe I deserve wonderful things?

Side of the Eye: What if my life continues to feel more positive?

Under the Eye: What if I can look back and notice how much has changed?

Under the Nose: What if the better I feel, the better my life gets?

Chin Point: I like these thoughts a lot.

Collarbone: These thoughts feel so much better.

Under the Arm: These thoughts feel good and maybe even a little more possible.

Top of the Head: What if feeling good really will draw more and more good to me?

Take a Breath.

You can tap on this sequence anytime you feel impatience surfacing.

Always a Work in Progress

"You are allowed to be both a masterpiece and a work in progress, simultaneously." ~ Sophia Bush

I often share with clients my own foibles in life. My foibles are always there, reminding me to keep tuning myself up—because I can get out of tune.

I have a dear friend who is my accountability buddy and we sometimes get a chuckle with each other when either of us will ask the other, "Hey, did you tap on that?" I do this for a living and I need to remind myself that any issue that surfaces is better met with tapping to relieve the stress first so you can get a fresher perspective on how to best handle the challenges in life. This may sound strange coming from someone who works with people with tapping, but I recommitted myself to tap daily, even if nothing challenging is going on and I see the cumulative effect of this.

Sometimes I notice more profound releasing than others, and I feel grateful to have this tool, at my fingertips, to help me along my journey in life.

When you think about tapping as a tool always available to you to assist you in your life, you become less afraid of your thoughts and emotions. You are not as stressed by your own internal negativity. You understand that you came by this thinking early in life, having these thoughts are natural.

Like I said before, I believe we come into this world filled with possibility and we learn to forget, early on, who we are and the world of possibilities within us. Tapping helps to restore your belief in yourself and what is possible for you. Over time with a consistent practice of tapping, I believe you will find you feel good about yourself more often, catch yourself quicker when headed down a rabbit hole of dysfunction, feel more peaceful and hopeful in life, release self-sabotage, and release a host of mental, emotional and physical health challenges.

And tapping has no known negative side effects.

233

I always let clients know that powerful emotions can occur while tapping, and this may feel like a downside—it is not. It means you have targeted stuck emotion and it's coming up to move out. It feels intense when it's being released, but if you keep tapping, you will feel soothed.

This brings me to a quote from Janice Berger's book I mentioned earlier, *Emotional Fitness: Discovering Our Natural Healing Power:*

"Feelings aren't buried dead. They're buried alive."

When strong emotion surfaces, realize this is a good thing and keep tapping so you can process this emotion through to its completion. If you keep tapping, you will get to the other side. Sometimes we cannot because we have blind spots, which is why it may be beneficial to get help from a trained professional. I also recommend you get help from a trained professional for using tapping for more emotionally charged issues. I will talk about this more at the end of this book.

Remind yourself that you are a work in progress and always will be. You will never do it all. As soon as you reach a new place, you will look for the next thing. You live in an evolving universe and you will always evolve.

You are an unfinished work in progress. One of the wonderful things about life's challenges:

"You get to find out that you're capable of being far more than you ever thought possible." ~Karen Salmansohn

234

Chapter Summary

Tapping can now be a tool, in your toolbox, that you can use anytime and anywhere that works for you, to create consistent lasting change.

Knowing you will always be a work in progress, helps to free you from feeling that there's some intended finish line you will cross over and be complete.

I find acknowledging that personal changes to improve yourself and your life, is a lifelong process we will never get done. We can find completion in many tasks, goals, or intentions we have for ourselves. But, inevitably, something more takes its place as the process continues.

Life is not static. As long as you're alive, you're going to either grow or regress, and if you're reading this book, I'd say you're someone who's seeking growth and with growth comes both things we move through with more ease and things that can trip us up.

Tapping is an effective tool to help you move through the things that have the potential to trip you up, so you can move forward with more ease.

It's always there to help you when you need it. Keep it in your toolbox and I believe you'll find your life unfolds in a way you feel empowered about along with leading you toward inspired action. Help is literally at your fingertips.

Conclusion

"The emotion that can break your heart is sometimes the very one that heals it..." ~ <u>Nicholas Sparks</u>, <u>At First Sight.</u>

Tapping can be a profoundly effective tool to help you embrace all parts of your emotions, even those you learned to reject; the forbidden ones. All of your emotions have an amazing life in them. They are rich with information, and there is good in every emotion you feel.

It is helpful to remind yourself there are no good or bad emotions. Emotions are indicators of where you are. The ones that feel negative are there to awaken you to your inner world and let you know that you embrace the limiting beliefs you learned.

Remember that it is not the emotion itself that is good or bad; it is the actions that can come from suppressed emotions that cause the real problems in your life.

As you embrace all of your emotions, you learn to not fear your emotions so intensely. You become the observer of your fear and what brings it on. With tapping, you have a tool to move through your emotions and feel them through to completion. When you complete an emotion, when you feel it through to the end, it no longer gets buried alive in you. Without the buildup of emotions, you become a clearer channel for your creative mind to be more readily accessible to you. This helps you to foster self-trust and to be true to yourself and your vision for your life. It opens you to guidance and direction that can make your life better. It also elevates your self-confidence.

You were born with this amazing palette of emotions installed within you. They are in you for a reason. If you still believe you shouldn't feel certain emotions, then it begs the question: Why would you have these emotions, if you are not supposed to feel or use them to help you?

Think about the organs in your body. You can live without some—although you will need to adjust compensate for the missing organs—yet they are there for a reason. When your body is functioning well, you are using all of your organs.

I see this time and time again with myself and my clients. When you accept your emotions, you use them to help get yourself back on track or keep you on track, and this allows you to open to the life that wants to come through you.

What now? Where do you go from here?

I recommend going back and doing the tapping exercises in this book as often as you need to. You will know when you are complete with them because the exercises do not land for you anymore. They will probably feel boring to you.

If you want to learn more about tapping and how to incorporate it into your life, please visit my website at www.martimurphy.com. There are many resources there for you. There's a complimentary download called How to End the Cycle of Failing and a complimentary 21 Days of Tapping Practice.

With the tapping practice download, you will receive a tapping script in your inbox every day for 21 days you can tap along with. There's also a money program complimentary Your Mindful Money Makeover at

https://yourmindfulmoneymakeover.com.

If you are interested in working more closely with me one to one, I invite you to contact me for a free consultation. Click here to book your complimentary Get-To-Know-You Session.

I also have a weekly on-line class, called Embrace, I run with a group of amazing people, if group work speaks to you. You

237

can learn more about this on my website or in the Get-to-Know-You-Session.

The session is available at no charge because I need to make sure we are a good fit to work together. Before you spend your time and resources in endeavoring on this tapping journey, make sure it feels like a fit for you too.

If you are looking for an EFT practitioner, interview all potential practitioners. You want to be sure you feel confident and safe with the person with whom you work. Before you begin work, be sure you can move on if anything does not feel right once you have started.

It is important when going to work on highly charged emotional circumstances that your trust is built during the first conversation with the practitioner. When interviewing someone to work with you, you should feel comfortable knowing you may leave without censure if it does not work out. You may need to ask about this.

I will add that if you notice a pattern within yourself of always leaving practitioners when headed into deeper emotional terrain, then that is worth looking at. You will know if you are afraid to go deeper or if it feels like it is not a fit to work together once you check in with yourself. This is good to remember.

This is very personal work, so you want to be sure that whatever choice you make, it feels light to you. When you are first learning to trust yourself and your feelings, I find using light and heavy to be helpful. Check in with whether it feels light or heavy in your body. The question to ask when deciding about any person, product or program is:

Does doing this feel light or heavy?

It is a great way to weigh in without having to be clear about what you are feeling. If you are not sure, you may need to ask more questions.

Your emotions are there for you, to help you, to guide you, to work in harmony with you. When you see them in this way, amazing possibilities open up for you.

I hope this book has helped you move forward to opening to the life that wants to come through you. I recommend you read it multiple times as you're a different person each time you do, and new things will stand out for you because you're ready to receive them. I wish you the best on your healing journey through your emotional landscape. I wish for all of your emotions to become available for you to feel without fear or feeling forbidden to you.

"The best and most beautiful things in the world cannot be seen or even touched. They must be felt with the heart." ~ Helen Keller

---

Acknowledgements

I would like to thank Irene Jorgensen for all of your rewrites and editing help. You have been a blessing and a gift to me on this journey with your wisdom, knowledge, and generosity of spirit.

I would like to thank my daughter Bailey for moving forward with this and your honesty in the process. To book editor Jamie Gifford for your edits and help with this book.

To Tammi Metzler, my book writing coach, for your vision and organization in helping me to make sense out of the book that was longing to come out.

Thank you to Slava my web person for being an absolute delight to work with and helping to create a website page that reflects the writings in this book. We are a team and you contribute so much.

To Joan Frantschuk for the following your intuition and creating a cover that reflects the writing.

To Joe Broadmeadow. You have been a priceless help to me in the publishing of this book. I'm truly grateful.

To anyone who has been in my life in any way that has been a help, support, and teacher to me through this life's journey.

To my parents Jim and Gloria for being two of my soul's greatest teachers. To my sister Mary for being the best person I've known in this lifetime. To my sisters Sarah and Susie for the family journey we continue to navigate through while loving each other even when things get sideways.

Last but not least, to my husband Liam who has without

question been a teacher and a revealer to me on my healing journey. To my daughter Bailey who has added so much goodness to my life and who fuels my desire to continue on this path of healing and helping. To my stepdaughter Quincy, who has been such a welcomed and wonderful addition to my life. To Charlie. You too were a great teacher, a friend and family all in one.

I have learned so much through the melding of our family. I love you all.

About Marti Murphy

I was always the good girl. The good employee. The responsible and reliable one.

And I was suffocating; I was quietly desperate.

On New Year's Eve of 2010, everyone was out partying, and I was at home pondering how another year had passed and nothing in my life had changed.

That was my decision point. My life sucked, and I knew I had to change things.

I set the intention to the universe, God, The Great Spirit. One of two things had to happen: if there was something out there that would help me change my life, that I would find it, and if not, then I just wanted peace with my mediocre life.

Two weeks later, I found EFT.

I found the "thing" that would change my life and change my life it did and continues to.

Fast forward to my life now.

I left my corporate career and started a personal transformation business.

I'm an Emotional Fitness Coach, Certified EFT Practitioner, and former host of the EFT Radio Show "From Ranting to Raving." I'm starting up a new local radio show in the town I live in on KUPR 99.9 FM.

I specialize in assisting my clients to clear their conflicts in their personal and business lives so they can create what they want.

For more information, please email me at marti@martimurphy.com.

References

Albrecht, S. (2017) Psychology Today, titled "The Psychology of Road Rage: Anger and Violence Behind the Wheel": Posted Jan 09, 2017, © 2019 Sussex Publishers, LLC

Berger, J. (2000) Emotional Fitness - Discovering Our Natural Healing Power (Penguin Canada: Penguin Group), page 13.

Canfield, J. (2019). Using the law of attraction for joy, relationships, money & success. Retrieved from https://www.jackcanfield.com/blog/using-the-law-of-attraction/

Church, D., Yount, G., & Brooks, A. J., (2012). The effect of emotional freedom techniques on stress biochemistry: A randomized controlled trial. The Journal of Nervous and Mental Disease, 200(10), 891-896.

Dispenza, J. (2009). Can you change your brain by thinking differently [Web log post]. Retrieved June 30, 2019 from https://drjoedispenza.net/blog/can-you-change-your-brain-by-thinking-differently/

Kline, F and Fay, J. (1990) Parenting with Love and Logic (NavPress, Colorado Springs, CO)

Hampton, D. (2016). How your thoughts change your brain, cells, and genes [Web log post]. Retrieved July 1, 2019 from https://www.huffpost.com/entry/how-your-thoughts-change-your-brain-cells-and-genes_b_9516176?

Part of HuffPost Wellness ©2019 Verizon Media. All rights reserved.

Hicks, E. (2004). Ask and It is Given: Learning to Manifest

Your Desires, New York: Hay House, Inc., p.114)

Lipton, B. (2012, June 7). The wisdom of your cells. Retrieved from https://www.brucelipton.com/resource/article/the-wisdom-your-cells

McTaggart, L. (2007). The intention experiment: Using your thoughts to change your life and the world. New York, NY: Simon and Schuster.

Moorjani, A. Interview by Evelyn Einhaeuser, Stories of Healing: Anita Moorjani: Dying to Be Me
Retrieved from http://www.synergies-journal.com/healing/2015/3/30/nmxa7sshsqba0gtjwd2jkqlnxy e1dg

Oppenheimer, M. (2008) The Queen of the New Age, New York Time Magazine May 4. 2008

Ordinary People. Directed by Robert Redford, performance by Mary Tyler Moore, Wildwood Enterprises, Inc, 19 September 1980

"Psychosomatics" Merriam-Webster.com. 2011. https://www.merriam-webster.com (8 May 2011).

Shapiro, D. (2002) The Body Mind Workbook: Vega 64 Brewery Road, London, N7 9NT, p. 154

Silver, T. (2019). Tosha Silver. Retrieved from https://toshasilver.com/

Tolle, E. (1999). Practicing the Power of Now: Essential Teachings, Meditations, and Exercises from the Power of Now. CITY, California: New World Library.

"Triggered" Collins English Dictionary - Complete & Unabridged Digital 2012 Edition © William Collins Sons & Co. LTD. 1979

Vanzant, I. (2016) An interview by Oprah Winfrey, Super Soul Sunday, 18, April 2016

Additional References

Schwartz, R. and Sweeney, M. Internal Family Systems (IFS) https://selfleadership.org.

Kootenay Columbia College of Integrative Health Science in Nelson, British Columbia, Canada

End Notes

——————————————

[1] Church, D., Yount, G. & Brooks, A. (2012). The Effect of Emotional Freedom Technique EFT on Stress Biochemistry: A Randomized Controlled Trial. Journal of Nervous and Mental Disease, 200(10), 891–896.

[2] https://www.dictionary.com/e/slang/triggered/

[3] *Ask and It Is Given: Learning to Manifest Your Desires,*" by Esther Hicks and Jerry Hicks Penguin Random House Publisher Services 2004

[4] Practicing the Power of Now, Eckhardt Tolle New World Library; 1 edition (September 2001)

[5] *www.eftuniverse.com*

[6] published at counsellingresource.com November 8th, 2011

[7] http://emofree.com/